Katholieke Universiteit Leuven
Groep Biomedische Wetenschappen
Faculteit Geneeskunde
Departement Neurowetenschappen
Laboratorium voor Cognitieve Neurologie

Functional specialisation within the language network: Effects of cortical dysfunction

Mathieu VANDENBULCKE

<u>Jury</u>:

Promotor:	Professor R. Vandenberghe, KUL
Voorzitter:	Professor W. Robberecht, KUL
Secretaris:	Professor W. Vanduffel, KUL
Leden:	Professor P. Agostinis, KUL
	Professor F. Maes, KUL
	Professor C. Price, University College London
	Professor E. Salmon, Université de Liège

Leuven, 01-02-2007

Doctoraal proefschrift in de medische wetenschappen

Foto cover : Toren van Babel (1563) door Pieter Breughel de Oude.

A CIP-record for this book is available from the Library of Congress.

ISBN 978-90-429-1938-9

Functional specialisation within the language network: Effects of cortical dysfunction

Mathieu Vandenbulcke, MD
Promotor: Rik Vandenberghe, MD, PhD

Dankwoord

Mijn oprechte dank gaat in de eerste plaats uit naar mijn promotor, Prof. Rik Vandenberghe. Ik heb het voorrecht om als eerste doctorandus onder zijn hoede te promoveren. Ik kan me geen betere promotor inbeelden. Hij liet ruimte voor zelfontplooiing maar stuurde bij waar nodig. Hij werkte inspirerend en motiverend. Tijdens onze wekelijkse overlegmomenten, kreeg ik les in logica en kritisch denken. Als uitmuntend en gerespecteerd wetenschapper introduceerde hij me in een wereld die ik anders nooit had leren kennen. Ik dank Prof. R. Vandenberghe voor deze zeer verrijkende jaren en hoop van harte dat deze de basis mogen vormen voor een verdere aangename en vruchtbare samenwerking.

Dank ben ik ook verschuldigd aan Prof. Paul Igodt en Prof. Koen Demyttenaere, respectievelijk uittredend en huidig diensthoofd van de dienst psychiatrie UZ Leuven. Ze hebben mij de kans gegeven om een eigen weg te bewandelen. Zo kon ik me wetenschappelijk en klinisch bekwamen in ouderen- en neuropsychiatrie, mijn voorliefde binnen het domein van de geestelijke gezondheidszorg. Veel medewerkers van onze dienst psychiatrie ben ik dankbaar voor hun vriendschap. Ook Dr. Jules Janssens, neuropsychiater, ben ik erg erkentelijk.

Ik wil ook de fysici danken met wie ik heb mogen samenwerken, met name Dr. Ronald Peeters en Prof. Patrick Dupont. Als pure wetenschappers met een open geest en onbaatzuchtige ingesteldheid verdienen zij het grootste respect. Maar vooral hun vriendschap heeft me erg veel deugd gedaan.

Ik denk nog vaak aan mijn sympathieke labogenoten en brothers in arms, Pascal, Leen, Katrien en Natalie. Ik heb zeer veel geestige herinneringen aan ons eiland maar apprecieerde evenzeer de rust en ingetogenheid. Ook Kathleen Porke en Carine Schildermans hebben mij vaak geholpen, waarvoor dank.

Dit klinisch werk was niet mogelijk geweest zonder de verwijzende neurologen en psychiaters, Dr. F. Bouckaert, Dr. I. Dehaene, Dr. T. Michielsen en Dr. M. Van Orshoven.

I am grateful to the members of my jury, Prof. P. Agostinis, Prof. F. Maes, Prof. C. Price, Prof. E. Salmon and Prof. W. Van Duffel for their insights, suggestions and comments.

De belangrijkste bijdrage werd ongetwijfeld geleverd door de patiënten en hun families. Ik besef heel goed dat ons onderzoeksprotocol een serieuze inspanning vroeg en bewonder hun geduld en medewerking. Zij gaven dit werk een zeer persoonlijk karakter en motiveren me elke dag om verder te zoeken. Ook het engagement van de vele oudere vrijwilligers die deelnamen aan dit project is echt bewonderenswaardig.

Mijn grootste waardering gaat uit naar mijn familie. De wetenschappelijke interesse van mijn moeder en haar inzet voor patiënten zijn voor mij altijd een voorbeeld geweest. De mensenkennis van mijn vader vind ik in geen enkel leerboek terug. Zijn humor en relativeringszin koester ik. Ook mijn schoonouders dank ik voor hun warmte en inzet voor hun (klein)kinderen.

Er is zoveel waar ik mijn broer, Luc, voor zou willen danken. De wetenschap dat er midden op zee, aan de andere kant van de wereld of in Antwerpen een hart op hetzelfde ritme klopt als dat van mij, is zo geruststellend.

Om mijn dank en liefde aan mijn echtgenote, Martine, te betuigen, zou een thesis niet volstaan. Martine, je bent de mooiste persooon die ik ken, voor Sophie en Victor ben je de liefste moeder die ik me kan inbeelden, je maakt me echt gelukkig, ik hou van je.

Afasie

Afasie
Afasie noemen wij het
Al is het erg:
de woorden vallen naast mij uiteen.
In het rond dansen zij.
Vaak speel ik met de letters;
Het blijkt dat de ernst niet in de letters zelf ligt, tot niemand er nog iets van
Begrijpt.
Onze gewichtige tante spraakkunst regeert
Terwijl nonkel
Borrelt met de losgeslagen
Letters
Spoortjes van de guitige boekstaven rollen over het lettertapijt
En
Zingen spraakonzinnig uit het repertoire van mijn hersens machine.
De ommekant
Is wel anders
Ik kan het niet
verletteren
Ik kan het niet
verwoorden
Noch verzinnen.

Dit gedicht werd geschreven door een patiënt met primaire progressieve afasie die deelnam aan deze studie. Dank U wel.

Contents

Chapter 1

Introduction

Behavioral studies of patients with cortical dysfunction and functional imaging studies in cognitively intact subjects are two key sources of evidence that have contributed to our knowledge about the neural architecture of language [1] [2] [3]. Patient studies and functional imaging studies in healthy subjects provide complementary information: Studies of patients with cortical damage indicate which regions are critical for a given function but rarely respect functional boundaries. Functional imaging studies achieve a superior spatial and cognitive resolution and allow one to study the intact brain directly, but it does not reveal which areas are critical, only which are more active. We took advantage of the complementary information provided by both approaches [4] to gain insight in the functional anatomy of language and semantic processing. We combined detailed neuropsychological and psychophysical examination with structural and functional imaging in patients and in healthy controls.

1.1 Aim of the thesis

The purpose of this thesis was twofold:

Our first aim was to test a model of functional anatomy of language and semantic memory. We determined the neuroanatomy of the associative semantic system [5] in normal elderly subjects. We examined how the different cortical components of this system contribute to language and semantic processing by studying the behavioral effects of cortical dysfunction in patients.

Our second goal was to gain insight in the pathogenesis of cognitive dysfunction in patients with neurodegenerative disorders. The two most prevalent cortical neurodegenerative disorders are Alzheimer's disease (AD) and frontotemporal lobe degeneration (FTLD). We focused on patients with primary progressive aphasia (PPA) [6], the language variant of FTLD [7], and patients with amnestic mild cognitive impairment (MCI) [8], a pre-dementia stage of AD. PPA and MCI have dissociable patterns of cognitive impairment. Patients with PPA experience progressive language dysfunction with relative preservation of episodic memory. Conversely, patients with MCI exhibit episodic memory problems with clinical preservation of other cognitive domains such as language. This allowed us to study neural changes associated with language impairment in PPA and to examine subclinical alterations within the language network in MCI.

1.2 Experimental model

Classical well-known language areas in the left hemisphere are Broca's area [9], located in the left inferior frontal gyrus (Brodmann's areas (BA) 44 and 45), and Wernicke's area [10], located in the posterior third of the superior temporal gyrus and sulcus and the middle temporal gyrus [11]. These areas have been identified more than a century ago on the basis of post-mortem studies and correlations with gross deficits that existed prior to demise [12]. Broca aphasia is characterized by impaired motor programming of speech and agrammatism among other deficits, whereas individuals with Wernicke aphasia experience a severe disruption in their ability to match words to their meanings [13].

More recent developments, such as in vivo structural brain imaging and in vivo imaging of brain function, have allowed it to refine the classical model and to reveal brain regions that are critically involved in language and knowledge processing beyond the classical perisylvian language areas (for a comprehensive review, see [14]). In an early PET study, we examined the neural substrate of associative-semantic judgements with words or pictures in healthy subjects [5]. We made a distinction between input-modality independent and input-modality specific areas. Input-modality independent areas are activated during associative-semantic judgements irrespective of stimulus presentation, words or pictures. Input-modality specific areas are activated during associative-semantic judgements with either words or pictures.

Based on findings from this original PET study [5] and other studies in healthy subjects, we proposed the following model of functional anatomy of language and semantic memory at the onset of this project in 2002:

- The posterior third of the left superior temporal sulcus and the left inferior frontal sulcus are word-specific areas [15] [5] [16] [14] [11]. These areas serve as gates of entry from the internal representation of a word into the semantic system [5].
- The left middle temporal gyrus is an input-modality independent associative semantic area [5] involved in the processing of a-modal semantic representations [17] [18] [19].
- The anterior and the medial temporal cortex function as associative structures that bind together representations of meaning that are distributed over human cerebral cortex [20] [5] [21].
- The left posterior inferior temporal gyrus (BA 37) is involved in linking a visual object [22] [23] [24] to the internal representation of its name [25] [26] [16].
- The posterior end of the left inferior temporal sulcus is a picture-specific area [5] and functions as a gate of entry from the internal representation of a visual object [27] [23] [28] into the semantic system [5].
- The dorsolateral prefrontal cortex is involved in searching the semantic "web" [5] and in short-term verbal memory [29] [30].

1.3 Patient populations

As mentioned above, we included patients with PPA and MCI to study the disease mechanisms underlying cognitive dysfunction in patients with neurodegenerative disorders. Patients underwent structural and functional imaging together with neuropsychological examination twice: At time of inclusion and after one year of follow-up. We included a third group of patients with ischemic lesions following stroke.

1.3.1 Primary progressive aphasia

Primary progressive aphasia is a syndrome of declining language function [31] [32] [33] [7] [6] [34]. PPA patients complain of word-finding difficulties, word comprehension problems or motor speech disturbances. The clinical diagnosis of PPA is made when other mental faculties such as memory for daily events, non-verbal episodic memory, visuospatial skills and comportment are relatively preserved, when language is the only area of salient and progressive dysfunction for at least the first 2 years of the disease, and when brain imaging does not show a specific lesion other than atrophy that can account for the language deficit [35].

Typically a distinction is made between progressive non-fluent aphasia (PNFA) [31] [6] [35] and semantic dementia (SD) [32] [33] according to fluency of speech and presence or absence of word comprehension problems [7]. Patients with PNFA present with impairment of spontaneous speech with phonemic paraphasias, neologisms, articulatory disturbances and agrammatism. Patients with SD exhibit disproportionate anomia in combination with single word comprehension difficulties and object recognition problems. The terms primary progressive aphasia and semantic dementia also have different origins [36]. Patients with semantic dementia have been classified on the basis of detailed *neuropsychological* assessments which revealed non-verbal as well as verbal semantic processing deficits [32] [33]. PPA on the other hand emphasizes the *clinical* presentation and the continuum between and within individuals [6]. Other subtypes, such as pure progressive dysarthria [37] or logopenic progressive aphasia [38] have been described as well.

Neuroimaging studies have documented predominantly left-hemispheric frontotemporal atrophy and hypometabolism in PPA [39] [40] [41] [42] [43] [38] [44]. Left perisylvian atrophy is present regardless of clinical presentation [35] [45] [44]. Direct comparison of PNFA and SD reveals relatively more prefrontal atrophy in PNFA and relatively more left anterior temporal atrophy in patients with SD [44] [38]. Symptom-based approaches have established an association between severity of anomia and the degree of left anterior temporal atrophy [44].

Recent efforts to account for the clinical diversity in PPA have focussed on the correlation between clinical presentation during life and pathological examination post-mortem [46] [47] [48] [49]. These early findings support an association between presence or absence of tauopathy and the behavioral syndromes of progressive non-fluent aphasia and semantic dementia respectively [46] [47]. Genetic studies have been carried out in patients with frontotemporal lobe degeneration (FTLD). FTLD covers two major clinical syndromes: a language variant, i.e. PPA, and a behavioral variant called frontotemporal dementia [7]. In familial cases of frontotemporal lobe degeneration, presence or absence of tauopathy has been associated with different mutations on the same chromosome: In familial cases of tau-based pathological changes, mutations have been identified in the microtubule-associated protein tau gene (MAPT) on chromosome 17q21 [50] [51]. In a collaboration between the department of molecular genetics of the University of Antwerp and our memory clinic, a breakthrough has recently been achieved in familial cases of tau-negative ubiquitin-immunoreactive neuronal cytoplasmic inclusions with the identification of a mutation in the progranulin gene (PGRN), also on chromosome 17q21 [52] [53]. Preliminary efforts to identify clinical language differences between FTLD patients with MAPT and PGRN mutations suggest that patients with MAPT mutations exhibit more phonological deficits whereas the language deficit in patients with PGRN takes the form of semantic disturbances [54].

Two functional imaging studies of language and semantic memory have been conducted in patients with PPA. In a PET study, patients with semantic dementia exhibit neural activity decreases during associative-semantic judgments in the left posterior inferior temporal cortex [55]. In a mixed sample of PPA patients, components of the language network were activated to the same extent in patients as in age-matched controls during fMRI [45]. The only marked abnormality in these patients was greater neuronal activation during the performance of language tasks but outside the areas traditionally considered part of the language network [45].

1.3.2 Mild cognitive impairment

Whereas PPA starts with language decline, the onset of clinically probable Alzheimer's disease (AD) is characterized by episodic memory decline. Recently, AD-related brain alterations that precede the dementia stage have evoked a lot of interest. In memory-clinic based cohorts, a valid clinical approximation of this pre-dementia stage is "amnestic mild cognitive impairment" (MCI) [56] [57] [58]. Amnestic MCI is clinically defined by the presence of a subjective complaint of memory decline, corroborated by an informant, objective impairment of episodic memory on routine neuropsychological assessment and minimal impact upon instrumental activities of daily living (IADL) [59]. Other cognitive domains are relatively preserved [60] or only mildly affected, in which case the designation "amnestic MCI-multi-domain" has been proposed [59] [61]. In memory-clinic based cohorts, when criteria [8] [62] are strictly applied and alternative causes are rigorously excluded, amnestic MCI is associated with a 15% yearly conversion rate to probable AD over a 3- to 5-year period [8] [58]. Approximately 80% of patients clinically diagnosed with amnestic MCI convert to probable AD within six years [8] [59]. Anatomical [63] and neuropathological features are consistent with incipient AD [64] [65] [56] [66]. Abnormalities consist of a decrease of neurons [65] and tau aggregation in entorhinal cortex [67] [68], tau aggregation in cholinergic neurons of the nucleus basalis [66] and an increase of neuritic plaques in neocortical areas, including middle temporal gyrus [69].

The clinical condition of amnestic MCI provides us with a time window to study AD-related events that chronologically precede the dementia stage [56]. In clinically probable Alzheimer's disease (AD), word finding difficulties are frequent, even at an early stage [70] [71] [72] [73] [74]. According to detailed neuropsychological studies [75] [76] [77] [78] [79] [80] [81], the underlying problem is a degradation of semantic memory. Early changes within the associative semantic network of patients with MCI or early AD have not been studied yet. Instead, fMRI studies in amnestic MCI have focussed on episodic memory and on medial temporal volumes of interest

[82] [83] [84] [85] [86]. Medial temporal mnemonic effects, such as fMRI signal attenuation with stimulus repetition [84] or activity increases during intentional encoding [82] [83] [85], are affected in MCI. Functional MRI [87] and PET [88] studies of language and semantic memory in AD document activity decreases of posterior perisylvian areas [87] as well as recruitment of the non-dominant hemisphere [88].

1.3.3 Ischemic lesions

We studied in detail one patient with a right occipitotemporal lesion following stroke within the territory of the posterior cerebral artery [89]. We compared the performance of this patient with another patient who had a roughly symmetrical lef-sided ischemic lesion. Isolated infarctions of a superficial branch of the posterior cerebral artery are rare [89] and provide a unique opportunity to study the critical contribution of the lesioned area to a cognitive process of interest. The most common cognitive manifestations of occipitotemporal lesions are visual object agnosia [90] [91] [92], alexia without agraphia [93] [94], prosopagnosia [95] [96] and disorders of color cognition [97] [98]. Alexia without agraphia is caused by lesions of the left ventral occipitotemporal cortex [93] [94]. Prosopagnosia refers to the inability to recognize familiar faces and can appear in isolation especially when the occipitotemporal lesion is confined to the right hemisphere [95] [96]. Disorders of color cognition can affect color categorization, color-name association, and color-object association and are linked to left hemisphere damage [97] [98] [99]. FMRI studies of patients with occipitotemporal lesions have focussed on alexia caused by left-sided lesions [93] [100].

1.4 Experimental tasks

1.4.1 Neuropsychological battery

Our neuropsychological battery included only validated Dutch test versions. Language assessment comprised the entire Aakense Afasie Test (AAT) [101] (consisting of spontaneous speech assessment, token test, reading, writing, repetition, naming and language comprehension), the verbal association subtest of the Psycholinguïstische testbatterij voor de taalverwerking van Afasiepatiënten (PALPA) [102] [103], the Animal Verbal Fluency (AVF) test and the Boston Naming Test [104] [105]. Visuoperceptual and visuospatial processing were tested with the Object Decision task from the Birmingham Object Recognition Battery [106] and the Number Location test from the Visual Object and Space Perception Battery (VOSP) [107] respectively. We tested executive functioning by means of Trail Making Test (TMT) [108] and Raven's Colored Progressive Matrices [109]. Verbal and non-verbal episodic memory were examined with the Auditory Verbal Learning Test (AVLT) [110] [111] [112] and the Rey Visual Design Learning Test (RVDLT) [110]

1.4.2 Semantic knowledge retrieval

Knowledge of concrete items embraces a wide range of properties, from its appearance, the sounds that it makes, what it is used for, its origin or the category to which it belongs, the associations it evokes, and other types of information sometimes called encyclopedic [21]. This multifaceted knowledge is referred to as "semantic" or "conceptual" knowledge or semantic memory [113] [114] [115] [116] [117] [118] [119] [120] [121] [122] [123] [24] [124] [125]. Evidence for selective impairment of semantic memory came from neuropsychological studies in patients with semantic dementia [126], a progressive brain disease characterized by gradual loss of word retrieval and word comprehension caused by atrophy of the left anterior temporal lobe [127] [32] [41]. The anterior temporal lobe is one component of a more distributed left-hemispheric system that is activated during associative-semantic judgements with words or pictures [5].

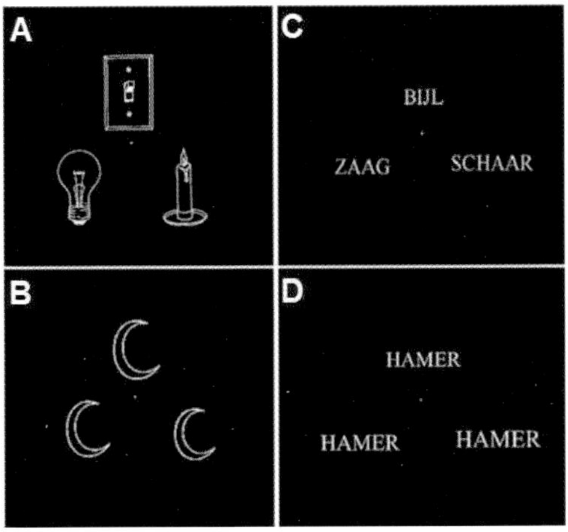

Figure 1.1: Stimuli and task. **A, C.** Associative semantic condition with pictures (*A*) or words (*C*). Subjects were instructed to press a left- or right-hand key depending on which of the two lower stimuli (test stimuli) matched the upper stimulus (sample stimulus) more closely in meaning. **B, D.** Associative semantic condition with pictures (*B*) or words (*D*). Subjects were instructed to press a left- or right-hand key depending on which of the two lower stimuli (test stimuli) matched the upper stimulus (sample stimulus) more closely in size.

In order to study the neuroanatomy of the associative semantic system in healthy elderly subjects and in patients, we adapted the original PET experiment [5] for use during fMRI. The design of the fMRI experiment was factorial (Fig.1.1) [5]. The first factor, task, had two levels: Associative-semantic (Fig.1.1*A,C*) versus visuoperceptual judgment (Fig.1.1*B,D*). The second factor, input modality, also had two levels: Pictures (Fig.1.1*A,B*) versus printed words (Fig.1.1*C,D*). The associative semantic condition (Fig.1.1*A,C*) was modified after the Pyramids and Palm Trees test [128] [32] [80]. Pictures were taken from the Snodgrass-Vanderwart set [129]. During a trial, a triplet of stimuli was presented for 5250 ms, one stimulus on top (the sample stimulus) and one in each lower quadrant (the test stimuli) (Fig.1.1), followed by a 1500 ms interval. Subjects had to press a left- or right-hand key depending on which of the two test stimuli matched the sample stimulus most closely in meaning. A given triplet was presented in either the picture or the word format and this was counterbalanced across subjects. In the visuoperceptual control condition (Fig.1.1*B,D*), a given stimulus was presented in three different sizes.

Differences between the original PET study and the current fMRI experiment included size of the stimuli: In the fMRI experiment, stimuli were presented at 3.8 deg eccentricity. Mean picture size was 5.6 deg and letter size 1.5 deg. In the original PET experiment, stimuli were presented at 6.7 deg eccentricity, mean picture size was 11 deg and letter size 3.2 deg. The smaller stimulus size in our fMRI experiment was necessary to match the size of the screen in the MR scanner. Second, the size difference in the visuoperceptual task between sample, target and distractor was 9 % in the fMRI experiment instead of 6 % in the original PET study. The intention of this adaptation was to anticipate decreased visuoperceptual discriminatory abilities in elderly subjects and patients. Third, the PET study included an extra condition in which subject had to make judgements about real-life size [130]. We dropped this condition in our fMRI experiment to limit the number of conditions in order to increase sensitivity. In contrast to the PET study, the fMRI experiment was applied only to elderly subjects (between 50 and 90 years) and many more healthy participants were scanned (37 versus 6).

The design of our fMRI experiment enabled us to probe the system for language and semantic memory and to study both modality-dependent (written words (see chapter 5) versus pictures (see chapter 6)) and modality-independent processes (see chapter 2 and 4). The distributed nature of the system mediating these processes [131] and the different cognitive functions fulfilled by the system's frontal [132] [133] and temporal constituents [18] are an advantage in this context: It allows one to probe multiple regions and multiple cognitive processes within one experiment. Our design did not include a low-level resting state condition as a reference because even the simplest baseline condition is associated with organized functional brain activity[134] which may itself be affected by disease [135]. Our factorial design also enabled us to account for performance differences by studying group-by-task interactions. Finally, to investigate disease-specific changes, one needs to apply the same paradigm across pathology. This necessitates a large control group of healthy elderly volunteers to match the different patient groups, making the use of multiple paradigms within one project impossible.

Based on neuropsychological observations in patients with selective impairment of knowledge of specific attributes, such as visual features [136] [137] [138] [139] [22] [140] or of specific categories such as biological entities [136] [113] [141] [142] [137] [138] [22] [139], different semantic subsystems have been proposed. Our fMRI paradigm did not allow us to investigate an attribute- or category-specific anatomical organization within the semantic system. For that purpose, we developed a battery consisting of oral feature generation, forced-choice naming to definition and free-hand drawing tasks (see chapter 6) to examine patients with lesions overlapping with the associative-semantic system. This battery was used only for behavioral testing.

1.4.3 Single word reading and object naming

Single word reading and object naming have evoked a lot of interest in language research (for reviews, see [143] [144]). Word reading shares many component processes with naming [16] [145] [146]: Retrieval of the internal representation of the word ("lexical" retrieval) [17] [18] [147] [148] [11] [149], retrieval of its meaning ("conceptual" or "semantic" retrieval) [150] [151] [21] [152] [153] and of what the word sounds like ("phonological" retrieval) [154] [155] [14] [156] [157]. Reading however differs from naming by the "gate" through which the knowledge system is entered and the path followed through the system [26] [16] [158] [24] [146]. Patients studies have contributed invaluably to our understanding of the cognitive architecture and neuroanatomical substrate of word reading and object naming (for reviews, see [159] and [160]). We developed different neuropsychological experiments to answer specific questions about both processes depending on the patient population.

To examine modality-specific identification deficits, we developed a chronometric experiment [161] [162] in which we presented words and pictures at different stimulus durations, including very short presentations (see chapter 5). We asked subjects to read the words or name the pictures. We only used single words that refer to concrete entities [163] [164] and we matched all concepts between pictures and words. Our chronometric analysis was based on a time-accuracy approach that allowed us to decompose word reading and picture naming into different processes [161] [162], including early visual identification and higher-order lexical processes. We developed this experiment to study word and picture processing with higher sensitivity in patients with MCI and to disentangle early visual identification problems from higher-order lexical processes. We related chronometric measures of word and picture identification to regional fMRI activity changes.

A second way to interfere with naming is to manipulate the context in which the picture must be named. In healthy subjects, retrieval of an object's name is facilitated by presenting a semantically related word (a prime) a few hundred milliseconds before picture onset [165] [166]. The prime propagates activity among word forms belonging to the same lexical-semantic fields and lowers the retrieval threshold for semantically related word forms [165] [167]. We applied a primed picture naming paradigm in patients with primary progressive aphasia. We studied whether impaired word retrieval in PPA results from impaired selection among competing neighboring word forms (see chapter 4).

A third factor that influences naming accuracy, apart from stimulus duration and context, is the semantic content of the picture. In patients with cerebral lesions, naming may be selectively impaired for objects belonging to a specific category, e.g. biological entities [136] [22] [141]. To examine category-specific naming deficits in patients with ischemic lesions, we conducted a confrontation naming experiment [168] in which subjects had to name 60 line drawings [129], covering three biological and three non-biological categories (see chapter 6). The stimulus set was matched between categories for frequency, visual complexity, familiarity, image agreement and prototypicality [129].

1.5 Imaging technique: Magnetic resonance imaging

1.5.1 General principles of MRI

Protons (i.e. the nuclei of the hydrogen atoms) give rise to most of the signal in an MR image. Protons have the property of "spin", i.e. they rotate around their main axis. The spinning protons combined with their net electrical charge create what is called a net magnetic moment, as if they were small magnets with a north and south pole. In the absence of any external magnetic field, the orientations of the proton magnetic dipoles are randomly distributed in the body. During magnetic resonance imaging, an external magnetic field, measured in tesla

(T), is applied by the scanner. Protons align either parallel or anti-parallel to the magnetic field, and the difference between these two populations gives the net magnetization vector. Protons do not align with external field in a straight line, but they precess or wobble around the axis of this magnetic field. The rate (or speed) at which the proton precesses is called the Lamor or precessional frequency and is proportional to the strength of the magnetic field. When a radiofrequency (RF) pulse at the Lamor (or precessional) frequency for hydrogen is applied, protons tilt away from the direction of the applied field. Once the pulse is terminated, the protons will start to relax and to attempt to realign again with the magnetic field. This process will take a finite period of time and will evolve with a time constant referred to as T1. As T1 occurs, another separate, but simultaneous phenomena called T2 occurs. This is the transverse relaxation time or T2 decay which is the natural decay of the signal in the transverse plane. Signals given out over the course of manipulations with RF pulses depend on the local microenvironment surrounding the proton. This property allows the signal obtained to be used to distinguish between different tissues in the body, or create *contrast*. The component of the imaging system that allows the spatial localization of the protons is a set of magnetic field gradients, set up by magnetic coils which are turned on and off.

1.5.2 Functional MRI

Blood flow, neural activity and BOLD response

Neuronal activity measurements are accompanied by changes in regional cerebral blood flow (rCBF) and blood volume (rCBV) due to changes in diameter of arterioles and venules as well as local capillary recruitment [169]. The best characterization of this hemodynamic response stems from optical imaging experiments [170] measuring changes in refraction of specific wavelengths of light. One component of this intrinsic signal originates from changes in blood volume and a second component from activity-dependent changes in oxygen saturation level of hemoglobin. These changes in saturation level result either from metabolic demands or from changes in blood flow affecting the relative amounts of hemoglobin and oxyhemoglobin. The time course of this hemodynamic response is well-known: When a neuronal population becomes more active, oxyhemoglobin concentration initially decreases, indicating an increase in cerebral metabolic rate of oxygen (CMRO2). However, after a few seconds, this decrease is reversed and after a further rise for 6 to 8 seconds the oxyhemoglobin concentration peaks. During this second phase of increasing oxyhemoglobin concentration blood flow exceeds what would be sufficient for the sole purpose of providing an active region with an increased demand of oxygen substrate ("uncoupling" between rCBF and oxidative metabolism) [171].

Changes of the concentration of oxyhemoglobin can be measured with magnetic resonance imaging (MRI). The magnetic state of the iron contained in the oxygen-carrying molecule hemoglobin is dependent on the amount of oxygen that is present in hemoglobin: Iron is paramagnetic when hemoglobin is depleted of oxygen (deoxyhemoglobin) and diamagnetic when the hemoglobin molecule is saturated (oxyhemoglobin). Changes of the relative concentration of oxyhemoglobin and deoxyhemoglobin induce local magnetic field changes and MRI signal changes. In functional magnetic resonance imaging (fMRI), MR imaging parameters are optimized to maximize the blood oxygenation dependency of fMRI signal. The thus obtained contrast is therefore called "blood oxygenation level dependent (BOLD) contrast. The BOLD response has been validated as a measure of hemodynamic response by combined fMRI and optical imaging [172]. Combined high resolution fMRI (in plane resolution of 0.75 x 0.75 mm) and microelectrode recordings in the primary visual cortex of the awake monkey provide evidence that BOLD contrast correlates well with local field potentials and thus with synaptic activity [171].

Image acquisition

The fast imaging technique of choice in functional magnetic resonance imaging sensitive to the BOLD contrast is echo planar imaging (EPI), a technique in which all the necessary information is generated from a single excitation. In EPI, the entire data set for a single plane is typically acquired in about 20-40 ms. For an fMRI experiment, the time interval between the RF pulse and the measurement of the middle echo (TE), i.e. the MRI signal, is about 40ms.

Optimization of acquisition

Multi-slice single shot EPI sequences suffer from distortion and susceptibility artifacts, especially in regions adjacent to air-holding cavities such as the anterior temporal lobe [173]. Given the importance of the anterior temporal lobe as a crucial component of the associative semantic system and its early degeneration in PPA [41] [44] [174] [175], we attempted to optimize the signal to noise ratio within this region [173]. Several less susceptibility sensitive acquisition sequences have been proposed but these sequences are also less sensitive to the BOLD contrast [176]. The solution used in this project, is a parallel imaging technique, called GeneRalized Autocalibrating Partially Parallel Acquisitions (GRAPPA) [177]. GRAPPA uses receiver coil arrays existing of a combination of a number of receiver coils (i.e. coils that capture the incoming signal), ranging from 2 to 32 elements. The spatial inhomogeneity and sensitivity of the separate elements is employed to decrease the number of acquired phase encoding steps for every separate coil element, by combining the different resulting images or raw data to one new reconstructed image [178] [179].

Procedural details

In all our experiments, echo-planar images were acquired using a 1.5 Tesla Siemens Sonata system (Siemens Medical Solutions, Erlangen, Germany) equipped with an 8-channel receive-only head coil (MRI Devices Corp., Waukesha, USA) with a TE/TR = 40/3000 ms and an acquisition voxel size of 3x3x3 mm^3. A single volume was obtained by acquiring 42 slices in the sagittal plane covering the entire cerebrum using the GRAPPA parallel imaging technique. Sagittal acquisition combined with GRAPPA maximizes sensitivity for anterior temporal activity changes and minimizes susceptibility artifacts [177].

Image analysis

Analyses of all our experiments were performed on data obtained from healthy elderly subjects and patients with neuro-degenerative disorders or patients with localized lesions. We used Statistical Parametric Mapping for image processing and statistics (Functional Imaging Laboratory, Wellcome Department of Imaging Neuroscience, London, UK), versions SPM99 and SPM02 as will be mentioned.

Data preprocessing

The EPI volumes from each subject were **realigned** using the first image as a reference for the purpose of removing movement between scans by use of an optimized procedure minimizing the residual sum of squares [180]. A mean EPI volume was obtained during realignment and **co-registered** with the structural MRI using mutual information processing [181].

The individual structural MRI's and EPI volumes were transformed so as to fit a standard template, a process called **normalization**. Variations in position and size are corrected by a 12-parameter affine transformation [180]; more subtle changes are corrected by a non-linear registration [180]..

Each point within the space into which brains are transformed is defined using three coordinates (in mm) [182]. The first coordinate defines the position in x, i.e. from left (negative) to right (positive) with 0 mm corresponding to the interhemispheric line. The second coordinate defines the position in y, i.e. from posterior (negative) to anterior (positive) with 0 mm corresponding to the anterior commissure. The third coordinate defines the position in z, i.e. from bottom (negative) to top (positive) with 0 mm corresponding to the plane through anterior and posterior commissure. The standard coordinate system allows us to express the localization of activations with respect to a fixed reference frame enabling comparisons between peak coordinates obtained in experiments from different laboratories.

After normalizing individual data these data are **smoothed** (i.e. convolved with a smoothing kernel). Smoothing individual images prior to a statistical analysis leads to an improved signal to noise ratio (SNR) provided that the width of the smoothing filter matches the size of the signal measured. Second, smoothing individual images improves overlap between activations obtained in different subjects. Indeed, between-subject variability in anatomical structure and functional organization may still be relatively large even after normalization to a standard template. Finally, smoothing conditions the data so that they conform more closely to a Gaussian field model as required by the theory of Gaussian Fields which lies at the basis of the correction procedure for multiple comparisons (cfr. below).

A statistical Parametric Mapping (SPM) analysis consists of two successive steps: First, a t statistic is calculated for each voxel and each contrast by use of massively **univariate** approach, then statistical inference is determined by use of **theory of Gaussian Fields**.

The general linear model

The first step of statistical analysis consists of linear multiple regression analysis [180]: The physiological measurement (or "response variable") in each voxel across scans and subjects is partitioned into a signal (or a set of "explanatory variables") as well as an error term. The explanatory variables are either part of the experimental manipulation or model noise in order to remove confounding effects of no interest from the error term. For each voxel parameter estimates express the contribution of each explanatory variable to the response variable. This contribution is estimated by use of the general linear model and standard least squares.

The general linear equation is:

$$x_{i,j} = g_{i,1}\beta_{1,j} + g_{i,2}\beta_{2,j} + ... + g_{i,K}\beta_{K,j} + \epsilon_{i,j} \tag{1.1}$$

where

- x is the response variable (physiological measurement)
- g is the explanatory variable (e.g. condition-specific effect)
- β is the parameter estimate
- ϵ is the error term
- i, ..., I indexes the observation (scan)
- j, ..., J indexes the voxel.

The general linear model decomposes the measurement in each voxel across scans into different components including the effect of each condition upon the measurement in this voxel. The contribution of different components is expressed in parameter estimates. We frame a regionally specific effect, i.e. a differential activation, in terms of a difference between parameter estimates for separate conditions in a given voxel. Such differences between parameter estimates are specified using linear contrasts between conditions. The significance of each contrast is assessed with a statistic with a Student's t distribution under the null hypothesis. For the purpose of facilitating comparisons between experiments and laboratories, the t-value is transformed to a Z score. The significance value for all voxels is comprehensively represented in a Statistical Parametric Map (SPM) map where each voxel is represented at its proper location on the brain template and where the Z value in this voxel for a given contrast is represented by use of a continuous color intensity code. At the second level, the individual Z maps are entered into a random effects analysis allowing inferences at population level. All contrast maps were submitted to an outlier and clustering detection analysis [183].

1.5.3 Structural MRI

Image acquisition

A T1-weighted structural volume was obtained by acquiring coronal inversion recovery prepared three-dimensional gradient echo images (MPRAGE: Inversion time = 800 ms, TE/TR 3.93/1950 ms, flip angle 12, 1 mm isotropic in-plane resolution) with a total acquisition time of 7 min 50 s.

Image analysis

Until recently, most in vivo quantitative assessment of patterns of brain atrophy were region-of-interest (ROI) based. However ROI measurements miss changes outside the ROI and thus may be inherently biased (in spatial terms). In addition ROI measurement errors are likely to be greater for structures with complex architectures, particularly if anatomical borders are defined by arbitrary criteria. The assessment may thus be subject to wide inter- and intra-rater variability. For this reason, ROI based morphometrics are difficult to replicate and compare between laboratories.

To avoid the constraints of ROI analysis, we used voxel-based morphometry (VBM) for the analyis of gray matter volume differences between subjects [184] [185] [186]. VBM is a fully automated whole-brain unbiased technique and has been validated in studies of degenerative dementias [186] [187]. We applied the optimized VBM protocol, as described by Good et al [185]. In the next paragraph, we will provide a brief methodological overview.

Before processing, the center point of all structural images was placed on the anterior commissure. For the normalization steps in chapter 2, 5 and 6, we used the standard MNI template implemented in SPM99 and SPM02. For the study described in chapter 4, we created an anatomical template based on 36 normal subjects (mean age 67.4 years, SD 7.9) imaged on the same MRI scanner with the same scanning parameters, in order to reduce any scanner specific bias and provide a template appropriate to the population samples. This involves spatially normalizing each structural MRI to the ICBM 152 template (Montreal Neurological Institute), using a 12 parameter affine transformation matrix. The normalized data are then smoothed with an 8-mm full-width at half-maximum (FWHM) isotropic Gaussian kernel, and a mean image (the template) is created. Separate grey matter templates were created by averaging all the smoothed normalized gray matter images.

The structural MR images (in native space) are segmented into gray and white matter images, followed by a series of fully automated morphological operations for removing unconnected non-brain voxels from the segmented images. The extracted segmented gray matter images are normalized to the gray matter templates thus preventing any contribution of non-brain voxels and affording optimal normalization of gray matter [184] [185]. However, the initial segmentation is performed on affine-normalized images (in native space), but the probability maps, used as Bayesian prior for segmentation, are in stereotactic space. Segmentation of fully normalized images is therefore preferable. In order to facilitate an optimal segmentation, the optimized normalization parameters are reapplied to the original, whole brain structural images (in native space) [185]. The optimally normalized whole brain structural images, which are now in stereotactic space, are then segmented into gray and white matter and CSF and subject to a second extraction of normalized segmented gray/white matter images. As a result of nonlinear spatial normalization, the volumes of certain brain regions may grow, whereas others may shrink. In order to preserve the volume of a particular tissue (gray matter, white matter or CSF) within a voxel, a further processing step is incorporated. This involves multiplying (or modulating) voxel values in the segmented images by the Jacobian determinants derived from the spatial normalization step [185]. In effect, an analysis of modulated data tests for regional differences in the absolute amount (volume) of gray matter. Each optimally normalized, segmented, modulated image is smoothed with a 12-mm FWHM kernel.

1.6 Imaging patients with brain disorders

1.6.1 Correlation between structural lesion and cognitive deficit

In neuropsychological studies, the interpretation of clinical manifestations associated with structural lesions raises a number of concerns. First of all, structural lesions do not respect functional boundaries. Second, functional reorganisation takes place in the lesioned brain. For instance, behavioral changes in patients with focal brain pathology do not necessarily imply a one-to-one structure function relationship. Behavioral deficits may arise as a consequence of functional changes in distant areas connected with the impaired area [55] [188]. For example, spatial attention deficits in neglect after right frontal damage correlate with abnormal activation of structurally intact parietal areas that mediate attentional operations in the normal brain [188]. Recovery of these attention deficits occur in parallel with restoration of activity in parietal areas. Another concern is that the absence of a behavioral deficit in the presence of lesion does not necessarily mean that the lesioned area is not involved in the process. Different brain regions may perform the same function, a phenomenon called degeneracy [189] [190] [191] [192] [4]. If only one system is lesioned, the cognitive function can be supported by the remaining degenerate system and performance will be maintained.

We solved these issues by combining structural and functional imaging studies in patients and in healthy controls. This allowed us to examine functional changes caused by disconnection and to uncover silent circuitries or compensatory mechanisms.

In neurologically impaired patients, it may be difficult to determine whether the dysfunctional brain region itself causes the impairment of a cognitive process or if the interaction with other regions [156] is responsible for the impairment. Changes in the interaction among brain regions are associated with task-dependent processing deficits, also called abnormal functional integration [4]. To explore this possibility, we used an extensive neuropsychological battery to evaluate cognitive processes under different task conditions. Second, the factorial design of our fMRI paradigm allowed us to investigate context-dependent functional impairment. Direct measures of functional integration, such as psychophysiological interactions (PPI) and dynamic causal modeling (DCM) examine how interactions among brain regions are modulated by experimental manipulations (effective connectivity). These analyses lay outside the focus of this project but are subject of future research in our laboratory.

1.6.2 Correlation between functional activity and cognitive deficit

In patient studies, the cognitive processes of interest are those that are impaired relative to normals [193] [194] [4]. If a process is impaired, how can the impaired process be activated to measure the neural correlates? The obvious approach is to engage subjects in tasks they can perform by making the task relatively easy and matching task performance between patients and controls. This approach allows one for *group comparisons* between patients and controls (see chapter 5). Another approach is to take advantage of the behavioral heterogeneity between patients and to *correlate* behavioral measures with brain activity [191] [192] (see chapter 2).

Normal task performance does not necessarily imply that all cognitive processes that lead to normal performance are intact. Intact performances in the presence of dysfunctional components of a brain system may reflect the use of different strategies to resolve the task, compensation by other components of the system or the fact that the system contains different components that fulfill the same function. Alternatively, activation in this area might reflect implicit or task irrelevant processing in healthy controls. However, it may be difficult to draw this conclusion from patient data. For instance, compensational mechanisms may be disease-specific. This means that an impaired area may cause behavioral deficits depending on the pathological circumstances. Second, behavioral deficits may be task dependent: Alternative strategies are more likely to be successful when the fMRI task is relatively easy. To uncover the critical contribution of dysfunctional areas in the presence of intact performance, one needs to combine a relatively easy fMRI task that probes a system with more sensitive psychophysical experiments that push the system to its limits (see chapter 5).

Another important issue in patient fMRI studies is the interpretation of activity changes outside the network activated by healthy controls, e.g. right hemisphere activation during language tasks after left-hemispheric stroke [195] [196] [197] [198] [199] [200] [201] [202] [203]. These activations may reflect compensatory activity in latent circuitries sustaining the same cognitive function [204] [190], changes in task-solving strategies [205], or maladaptive changes caused by deafferentation [206]. In stroke literature, it is still a matter of debate whether right-sided functional changes during language tasks are adaptive [195] [196] [202] [204] or not [197] [207] [208] and whether the adaptiveness is time- [198] or task-dependent [209] [210]. Interventional studies may reveal whether functional changes outside the network activated by normals are beneficial or detrimental. Different strategies exist: One can actively interfere with regional brain activity using transcranial magnetic stimulation [211] [212] [213]. Transcranial magnetic stimulation can transiently increase [213] or decrease [212] [211] cortical excitability depending on the stimulation frequency. Another interventional strategy is to train patients intensively and to correlate activity changes with measures of training-induced improvement [214]. These interventional strategies lay outside the scope of this project.

Patient fMRI studies also herald a number of technical concerns. In patient fMRI the major contribution to signal artifacts comes from bulk head motion during the acquisition of the functional series [215]. Two kinds of motion can be distinguished: Intra-image motion is generally very fast and sudden motion (i.e. at a time scale smaller than the image acquisition time) and inter-image motion on a time scale between a couple of seconds to minutes which is a slow movement of the subject. These two motion types have different effects on the acquired image and the functional map properties. Intra-image motion is typically induced by sudden head movements and results in ghosting artifacts in several slices of the acquired EPI volumes. When motion occurs perpendicular to the acquisition plane, it can also change the contrast in the images. Through plane head motion will result in a change of apparent repetition time for the acquisition of the same slice in different volumes. In other words the tissue has experienced a different "spin history". Our subjects were scanned with their head fixed in the axial plane by means of MRI compatible devices. We acquired sagittal slices during our experiment because we expected head motion from back to front in the sagittal plane. Inter-image motion leads to misregistration of the images within the time series and makes activation foci undetectable or induces artifactual activation when the movement is correlated to the stimulus. Correction for inter-image motion is achieved by realignment of the consecutively acquired images in the data series with the first image [216] [217] [181], as outlined in the section image analysis.

As outlined above, during preprocessing, individual brain images are transformed to standard space defined by a template image. As the template is typically derived from normal brains, nonlinear transformations can lead to inappropriate image distortion at the site of brain damage or inappropriate registration to the template [4]. One solution is to limit non-linear contributions. However, this negates the contribution of non-linear deformations which improves normalization both in healthy subjects and in patients [218] and was not applied in this project. Another solution is to mask lesioned areas and to exclude these areas from calculation of image differences in spatial normalization [218]. This approach may be of interest in patients with well-defined lesions, but does not apply to atrophic changes in patients with degenerative disorders. We adapted a pragmatic approach by using the normal procedure and inspecting the images visually to detect mal-registration.

Local brain atrophy may also influence regional cerebral activation [219] [220]. Spatial normalization may be insufficient to equalize group-differences in regional cortical volume [220]. Consequently, systematic anatomical variation indicative of specific subject population can contribute to between-group differences of functional activity. To exclude this confound, we performed between-group comparisons of gray matter volume (VBM) in areas where fMRI response differed between controls and patients. We are currently exploring more sophisticated methods to correct the fMRI signal for local atrophy [221].

BOLD signal depends on neurovascular (un)coupling. Neurovascular disruption may cause abnormalities even when neural activity is normal. There is no reason to assume that neurovascular abnormalities are context-dependent. Because fMRI responses equal activity differences between two conditions, activity changes due to abnormal neurovascular phenomena should be canceled out by subtracting the control condition from the active condition. In this project, we used group-by-task interactions instead of group comparisons based on a single task. Specific conditions that can cause abnormalities of neurovascular physiology include cerebral ischaemia, carotid stenosis, hypertension, diabetes mellitus, hypercholesterolemia and medication [222]. Rather than using these age-associated clinical conditions as exclusion criteria, we matched these risk factors between controls and patients.

1.7 Summary

We probed the system for language and semantic memory by means of a modified version of the Pyramids and Palm Trees test. This classical neuropsychological test of associative semantic memory calls upon both modality-dependent (written words versus pictures) and modality-independent processes. By studying the effect of cortical dysfunction, we examined the contribution of word-specific (see chapter 5), picture-specific areas (chapter 6) and modality independent areas (chapter 2 and 4) to language and knowledge processing.

We studied the pathogenesis of cognitive dysfunction in patients with neurodegenerative disorders. In chapter 2, we tested the hypothesis that, in analogy with other focal aphasic disorders, PPA would be associated with an activity shift toward right-hemispheric areas homotopic to the left-sided areas hit by the disease. In chapter 3, we studied the cognitive architecture of word-finding difficulties in PPA. In chapter 4, we determined the neural substrate of progression of language impairment in PPA. In chapter 5, we examined whether the language network is altered in amnestic MCI despite clinical preservation.

Chapter 2

Anterior temporal laterality in primary progressive aphasia shifts to the right

Annals of Neurology, 58, 362-370, 2005
Mathieu Vandenbulcke[1], Ronald Peeters[2], Paul Van Hecke[2], Rik Vandenberghe[1,3]
[1]Cognitive Neurology Laboratory, Section Experimental Neurology, K.U. Leuven, [2]Radiology Department, [3]Neurology Department.

2.1 Abstract

In aphasia due to stroke, language-related activity shifts towards right-sided areas homotopical to the left-sided lesion site. We examined whether a similar shift takes place in primary progressive aphasia (PPA). Nineteen PPA patients participated, together with 19 healthy subjects and 14 patients with amnestic mild cognitive impairment who served as controls. Subjects underwent neuropsychological assessment, structural magnetic resonance imaging (MRI) and a functional MRI with a factorial design: Words versus pictures and associative-semantic versus visuoperceptual task. Factor analysis of the neuropsychological data isolated 4 factors, with a cluster of language tests explaining the largest amount of total variance. Individual factor scores were entered as regressors into a regression analysis. Outcome variables were brain volume and response amplitude during the associative-semantic versus control conditions. Language competence correlated *positively* with volume and with responses in left anterior temporal cortex but *inversely* with responses in the right-sided homotope. In normals, anterior temporal activation was more extensive to the left than the right (laterality index (LI) 0.64 (s.e. +0.11). Laterality was inverted in PPA with word comprehension deficit (LI -0.34, s.e. 0.19), with an intermediate pattern in PPA without comprehension deficit (LI 0.23 (s.e. +0.14)). The rightward laterality shift previously reported in aphasic stroke extends to PPA.

2.2 Introduction

Recruitment of the un-affected non-dominant hemisphere is a robust finding in studies of the language system after stroke [195] [196] [197] [198] [199] [200] [201] [202] [203]. This contralesional activity is localized homotopically to the left-sided peri-sylvian lesion site, e.g. inferior frontal [198] [204] [223] or posterior temporal cortex [196] [198] [202]. This phenomenon has been observed as early as 24 hours following stroke [198] and has been described as a "laterality shift" [199]. A similar shift towards homotopical right-sided areas takes place in tumor patients with aphasia [224] [212]. We examined whether primary progressive aphasia (PPA), a focal neurodegenerative disorder [6] [43], is also associated with a laterality shift.

We combined voxel-based morphometry (VBM) with functional magnetic resonance imaging (fMRI) in PPA patients with or without single word comprehension deficit [6]. We included a healthy as well as a patient control group. The patients fulfilled the Petersen et al. (2003) criteria for amnestic mild cognitive impairment [62]. We adapted a classical neuropsychological test of associative semantics, the Pyramids and Palm Trees test [32] [128] [5], for use in fMRI. Compared to visuoperceptual judgments, this task activates a distributed left-hemispheric system that is common for words and pictures [5]. Given the focal nature of the symptoms associated with PPA, we tested the hypothesis that, in analogy with other focal aphasic disorders [196] [198] [202] [223], PPA would be associated with a shift of activity during the associative-semantic condition towards right-hemispheric areas homotopic to the left-sided areas hit by the disease.

2.3 Subjects and Methods

2.3.1 Subjects

Nineteen patients who fulfilled the criteria for primary progressive aphasia (PPA) [6] [43] participated, 10 men and 9 women, between 45 and 78 years of age (mean 68.6, s.d. 8.0 years), with a mean educational level of 12.3 years (s.d. 3.0) and a mean Oldfield score of +85.3 [225]. One PPA subject (case 13) was left-handed (Oldfield score -73). Word retrieval problems were the primary reason for attending the memory clinic in all patients. Language assessment comprised the validated Dutch version of the Aachen Aphasie Test, ("Akense Afasie Test", AAT) [101] and the verbal associative-semantic task of the validated Dutch version of the Psycholinguistic Assessment of Language Processing in Aphasia (PALPA) [102] [103].

In all PPA subjects, the score of at least one language task fell two standard deviations below the mean of control subjects (Table 2.3.1, 2.2). Seven out of 19 PPA patients (cases 1 to 7) scored 2 standard deviations below the mean of normal controls on the AAT word-picture matching tasks, both in the visual and the auditory modality, as well as on the PALPA verbal association task. This is indicative for a significant word comprehension deficit. These patients were also significantly more impaired on the Object Decision task (Birmingham Object Recognition battery [106]) than PPA patients without word comprehension problems (Table 2.3). Conversely, PPA patients without word comprehension deficit were significantly more impaired on the "articulation" and the "syntactic structure" sub-items of the AAT than those who had

	PPA			Controls	MCI	total
	SD	PNFA	all			
AAT						
Naming	**78.4*** (19.0)	**104.5** (12.0)	**94.9** (19.4)	116.7 (4.0)	114.5 (4.2)	/120
Comprehension						
Auditory word-picture matching	**18.4*** (4.1)	**24.2** (3.3)	**22.1** (4.4)	28.4 (2.1)	27.0 (2.7)	/30
Auditory sentence-picture matching	**25.1** (3.4)	**25.8** (3.7)	**25.5** (3.4)	29.3 (1.2)	28.2 (2.3)	/30
Visual word-picture matching	**19.2*** (6.0)	27.4 (2.5)	**24.4** (5.5)	28.9 (1.1)	28.5 (1.5)	/30
Visual sentence-picture matching	**24.6** (3.7)	**24.6** (2.2)	**24.6** (2.7)	28.2 (2.3)	27.9 (2.0)	/30
Total	**87.8*** (13.7)	**101.7** (9.4)	**96.6** (12.8)	113.7 (5.3)	111.7 (5.1)	/120
Token Test	**10.8** (11.8)	**7.0** (6.1)	**8.4** (8.6)	1.1 (1.9)	3.9 (5.3)	/50
Spontaneous speech						
Communicative behavior	**4.0** (0.8)	**3.7** (0.9)	**3.8** (0.9)	5.0 (0.0)	5.0 (0.0)	/5
Articulation	4.9 (0.4)	**4.1*** (0.6)	**4.4** (0.6)	5.0 (0.0)	4.9 (0.3)	/5
Automatized language	**4.1** (1.0)	**4.3** (0.5)	**4.3** (0.6)	5.0 (0.0)	4.9 (0.3)	/5
Semantic structure	**3.7** (0.7)	**3.9** (0.3)	**3.9** (0.3)	5.0 (0.0)	4.9 (0.3)	/5
Phonological structure	**4.6** (0.5)	**4.0** (0.7)	**4.2** (0.7)	5.0 (0.0)	4.8 (0.4)	/5
Syntactic structure	**4.3** (0.5)	**3.2*** (0.9)	**3.5** (0.9)	5.0 (0.0)	4.7 (0.5)	/5
Total	**25.4** (3.5)	**23.5** (3.5)	**24.2** (3.5)	30.0 (0.0)	29.3 (1.2)	/30
PALPA	**20.2*** (3.9)	26.7 (1.7)	**24.3** (4.1)	28.2 (1.8)	28.5 (1.4)	/30
Object Decision	**20.7*** (3.9)	24.7 (3.4)	23.2 (4.0)	27.1 (1.8)	24.7 (3.3)	/32
CPM	**21.7** (4.8)	**26.5** (5.0)	**24.7** (5.4)	31.6 (2.6)	29.7 (5.8)	/36
TMT	3.2 (1.5)	3.3 (1.2)	3.3 (1.3)	2.8 (1.0)	2.74 (0.66)	-
Number Location	9.0 (1.1)	9.2 (0.8)	9.1 (0.7)	9.5 (0.9)	9.1 (0.9)	/10
AVLT						
Learning	**24.2** (10.2)	35.8 (10.6)	31.5 (11.7)	49.0 (9.5)	33.7 (8.8)	/75
Recall	**3.5** (2.6)	8.2 (3.8)	6.4 (4.1)	11.0 (2.4)	4.2 (3.2)	/15
% Recall	**46.7** (25.9)	84.3 (16.3)	70.4 (27.1)	88.0 (10.5)	48.0 (26.7)	%
Recognition	**11.7** (1.1)	12.7 (1.6)	12.4 (1.5)	14.3 (1.4)	11.4 (3.6)	/15
RVDLT						
Recognition	13.2 (1.2)	12.5 (1.3)	12.7 (1.3)	13.7 (1.5)	11.2 (2.8)	/15

Table 2.1: Neuropsychological group data (mean (s.d.)). **Bold**: Significantly different between PPA and normals at $P \prec 0.05$ corrected for multiple comparisons. * : Significantly different between SD and PNFA at $P \prec 0.05$. *Abbreviations:* AAT: Akense Afasie Test. PALPA: Verbal associative-semantic test of the Psycholinguistic Assessment of Language Processing in Aphasia. Object decision: Object Decision test of the Birmingham Object Recognition Battery [106]. CPM: Raven's Coloured Progressive Matrices [109]. TMT: Time in sec during Trail Making Test part B divided by the time in sec during part A [108]. Number location: Number location test of the Visual Object and Space Perception Battery [107]. AVLT: Auditory Verbal Learning Test [111]. Learning: Sum of scores obtained on the 5 learning trials; Recall: Total number of items remembered after a 30 min delay; % recall: Number of items remembered after the delay divided by the number of items encoded. RVDLT: Rey Visual Design Learning Test [110].

word comprehension problems (Table 2.3). The AAT articulation sub-item measures articulation, prosody and speech flow (words per minute). Syntactic structure measures complexity and completeness of a sentence, word order, and usage of inflections and conjugations. An extensive neuropsychological protocol allowed us to exclude significant impairment in cognitive domains other than language in all PPA subjects (Table 2.3.1, 2.2).

Two control groups underwent an identical protocol:

1. Nineteen normal controls, matched for gender (10 men, 9 women), age (mean age 69.1, s.d. 8.7), educational level (12.3 years, s.d. 2.6), and handedness (Oldfield score +86.7) [225]. As in the PPA group, 1 control subject was left-handed (Oldfield score -64)

2. Fourteen patients who fulfilled the criteria for amnestic Mild Cognitive Impairment (MCI) [226], matched for gender (8 men, 6 women), age (mean 66.5, s.d. 7.0 years), handedness (Oldfield score + 89.6), and educational level (12.8 years, s.d. 2.7). One subject was left-handed (Oldfield score -46).

All subjects gave written informed consent in accordance with the Declaration of Helsinki. The study protocol was approved by the Ethical Committee, University Hospital Gasthuisberg,

Case	1	2	3	4	5	6	7	8	9	10	11	12	13	14	15	16	17	18	19	to
Age	59	64	69	70	73	74	74	45	57	65	66	68	71	72	74	74	76	77	78	-
Education	12	10	14	6	10	10	8	12	20	14	12	12	12	12	14	15	17	12	12	-
Disease duration	5	2	2	7	4	2	2	2	5	2	3	4	5	12	4	3	2	4	2	-
FAQ	**3**	**2**	**2**	**3**	**3**	**3**	**2**	**2**	**3**	**2**	**2**	**2**	**3**	**2**	**4**	**2**	**3**	**2**	**2**	/
BNT	**36**	**14**	45	**13**	**15**	**28**	**36**	**30**	53	44	52	**38**	**35**	46	**24**	56	**39**	43	**41**	/
AVF	**7**	**10**	14	**8**	**9**	**12**	**12**	**10**	18	17	17	23	**9**	**7**	**10**	23	**7**	**12**	17	-
AAT																				
Naming	**74**	**77**	**86**	**76**	**44**	**84**	**108**	**84**	109	**103**	117	112	**99**	114	**82**	117	**99**	**103**	116	/
Comprehension																				
Auditory word	**13**	**17**	**24**	**23**	**14**	**18**	**20**	**22**	30	28	22	**19**	28	**24**	**22**	27	**24**	**21**	**24**	/
Visual word	**10**	**22**	**26**	**22**	**12**	**19**	**24**	28	30	29	**21**	**25**	27	27	27	28	27	30	30	/
Auditory sentence	**26**	28	30	**25**	**19**	**24**	**24**	**20**	**29**	**23**	**25**	27	30	**26**	**18**	27	27	28	30	/
Visual sentence	25	28	27	25	**23**	**17**	27	**21**	27	**23**	26	26	27	**23**	**21**	25	24	26	27	/
Total	**78**	**95**	107	**95**	**68**	**77**	**95**	**91**	**116**	**103**	**94**	**97**	112	**100**	**83**	107	**102**	105	111	/
Token Test	**10**	1	2	**6**	**19**	**34**	4	0	**16**	**18**	**10**	1	3	1	**7**	0	**11**	**9**	**9**	/
Spontaneous speech	**26**	**29**	**23**	**26**	**26**	**19**	**29**	**20**	**21**	**27**	**28**	**28**	**22**	**26**	**21**	**22**	**19**	**20**	**28**	/
Phonological	**4**	5	**4**	5	5	**4**	5	**4**	**3**	**3**	5	5	**4**	**4**	**4**	**4**	**3**	**4**	5	/5
Syntactic	**4**	5	**4**	**4**	**4**	**4**	5	**4**	**3**	**4**	**4**	**4**	**3**	**4**	**2**	**3**	**2**	**2**	**4**	/5
Articulation	**4**	5	**4**	**4**	**4**	**4**	5	**4**	**3**	**4**	**4**	**4**	**3**	**4**	**2**	**3**	**2**	**2**	**4**	/5
Communicative	**4**	5	**3**	**4**	**4**	**3**	5	**4**	**3**	**3**	5	5	**3**	5	**3**	**3**	**3**	**3**	5	/5
Automatized	5	5	**4**	**4**	**4**	**2**	5	**4**	**4**	**4**	5	5	**4**	5	**4**	**4**	**4**	**4**	5	/5
Semantic	**4**	**4**	**4**	**4**	**4**	**2**	**4**	**4**	**4**	**4**	**4**	**4**	**4**	**4**	**4**	**4**	**3**	**4**	**4**	/5
PALPA	**22**	**24**	**21**	**22**	**12**	**19**	**22**	**24**	29	29	27	26	29	26	26	28	25	25	26	/
Object decision	**17**	**22**	27	24	**16**	**19**	**20**	**23**	30	22	**23**	**22**	27	26	25	32	**22**	**21**	24	/
CPM	**21**	**23**	30	**17**	**20**	**16**	**25**	28	31	32	**23**	28	**21**	27	**17**	35	29	**24**	**23**	/
TMT	2.9	2.2	2.9	**6.4**	2.3	3.6	2.3	3.0	**6.6**	2.2	2.9	2.5	3.4	3.5	2.4	2.1	3.1	4.0	4.1	-
Number location	10	9	10	10	9	8	7	10	10	9	9	10	10	10	10	9	8	8	8	/
AVLT																				
Learning	**15**	34	31	**10**	24	**18**	37	53	45	**24**	35	36	35	39	30	54	**19**	**29**	31	/7
Recall	**2**	**3**	**3**	**1**	1	6	**8**	15	**14**	**5**	7	8	10	7	7	13	**4**	**4**	**5**	/
% Recall	**40**	**43**	**30**	**33**	**16**	85	80	115	93	100	70	80	91	78	87	93	80	**50**	75	%
Recognition	13	15	14	**11**	14	13	13	14	**11**	12	12	13	13	12	15	14	**10**	14	12	/
RVDLT																				
Recognition	13	15	14	11	14	13	13	14	11	12	12	13	12	12	14	14	**10**	14	12	/

Table 2.2: Individual PPA patient data. *Bold:* 2 standard deviations lower than average of control group. Age and education in years. Case indices correspond to the numbers in Fig. 2.1. *Abbreviations:* FAQ: Functional Activities Questionnaire. AVF: Animal Verbal Fluency. Other abbreviations: See Table 2.3.1.

Leuven.

2.3.2 fMRI experiment: Stimuli and tasks

Stimuli were projected from a Barco 6300 LCD projector (1280x1024 pixels) onto a screen 28 cm in front of the subjects' eyes. The experiment was conducted using Superlab for PC version 2.0 (Cedrus, Phoenix, AR, USA).

The design of the fMRI experiment was factorial (Fig.1.1) and similar to that of a previous positron emission tomography study in healthy subjects [5]. The first factor, task, had two levels: Associative-semantic (Fig.1.1*A,C*) versus visuoperceptual judgment (Fig.1.1*B,D*). The second factor, input modality, also had two levels: Pictures (Fig.1.1*A,B*) versus printed words (Fig.1.1*C,D*). The associative semantic condition (Fig.1.1*A,C*) consisted of a modified version of the Pyramids and Palm Trees test [128] [32] [80]. During a trial, a triplet of stimuli was presented for 5250 ms, one stimulus on top (the sample stimulus) and one in each lower quadrant (the test stimuli) (Fig.1.1). Subjects had to press a left- or right-hand key depending on which of the two test stimuli matched the sample stimulus more closely in meaning. A given triplet was presented in either the picture or the word format and this was counterbalanced across subjects. In the visuoperceptual control condition (Fig.1.1*B,D*), a stimulus was presented in three different sizes. Subjects had to press a left or right-hand key depending on which of the two test stimuli matched the sample stimulus more closely in size on the screen. Two successive trials were separated by a 1500 ms interval. Each epoch, i.e. a block of trials of the

	PPA with	PPA without	
	comprehension deficit		
AAT			
Naming	**78.4** (19.0)	104.5 (12.0)	/120
Comprehension			
Auditory word-picture matching	**18.4** (4.1)	24.2 (3.3)	/30
Auditory sentence-picture matching	25.1 (3.4)	25.8 (3.7)	/30
Visual word-picture matching	**19.2** (6.0)	27.4 (2.5)	/30
Visual sentence-picture matching	24.6 (3.7)	24.6 (2.2)	/30
Total	**87.8** (13.7)	101.7 (9.4)	/120
Token Test	10.8 (11.8)	7.0 (6.1)	-
Spontaneous speech			
Communicative behavior	4.0 (0.8)	3.7 (0.9)	/5
Articulation	4.9 (0.4)	**4.1** (0.6)	/5
Automatized language	4.1 (1.0)	4.3 (0.5)	/5
Semantic structure	3.7 (0.7)	3.9 (0.3)	/5
Phonological structure	4.6 (0.5)	4.0 (0.7)	/5
Syntactic structure	4.3 (0.5)	**3.2** (0.9)	/5
Total	25.4 (3.5)	23.5 (3.5)	/30
PALPA	**20.2** (3.9)	26.7 (1.7)	/30
Object Decision	**20.7** (3.9)	24.7 (3.4)	/32

Table 2.3: Comparison between PPA patients with and without comprehension deficit (mean (s.d.)). Bold: Significantly different at $P \prec 0.05$.

same type, consisted of 4 trials (total duration 27 s).

Stimuli were presented at 3.8 deg eccentricity. The pictures were taken from the Snodgrass-Vanderwart set. Mean picture size was 5.6 deg and letter size 1.5 deg.

Performance of the fMRI tasks was analysed by means of a three-factor repeated-measures Analysis of Variance of reaction times, accuracies and omissions with stimulus modality and task as within-subject factors (two levels: pictures versus words and semantic versus visuoperceptual, respectively) and group as between-subject factor (three levels: PPA, MCI and normals).

2.3.3 Image acquisition

A 1.5 tesla Siemens Sonata system (Siemens Medical Solutions, Erlangen, Germany) equipped with an 8-channel receive-only head coil (MRI Devices Corp., Waukesha, USA) provided a T1-weighted structural volume (coronal inversion recovery prepared three-dimensional gradient echo images; Inversion time 800 ms, TE/TR 3.93/1950 ms, flip angle 12, 1 mm isotropic in-plane resolution) as well as T2* echo-planar images (EPI) (TE/TR 40/3000 ms). EPIs comprised 42 sagittal slices covering the entire cerebrum (voxel size 3x3x3 mm^3). Usage of the GeneRalized Autocalibrating Partially Parallel Acquisitions (GRAPPA) method maximized sensitivity for anterior temporal activity changes and minimized susceptibility artefacts [177].

A total of 116 volumes were acquired during each run. The first 8 volumes were excluded from analysis to allow for equilibration of the MR signal. Each run consisted of 3 replications of each of the 4 conditions. Subjects underwent 4 to 6 runs each.

2.3.4 Image analysis

We conducted two multiple linear regression analyses with individual neuropsychological factor scores as regressors and differences in brain volume and brain response amplitude, respectively, as dependent variables. We used Statistical Parametric Mapping 2002 for image processing and statistics (Functional Imaging Laboratory, Wellcome Department of Imaging Neuroscience, London, UK).

The individual factor scores were calculated as follows: Factors were extracted from the neuropsychological test scores of all 52 subjects using the eigenvalue one test (Henry F Kaiser) and orthogonal rotation (Statistica version 6, StatSoft, Inc, OK, U.S.). For each of the factors that had an Eigenvalue higher than 1, we calculated the individual factor scores. These individual factor scores express how well a given subject performs on the tests clustered by that factor. The individual scores of each significant factor were entered as regressors into a multiple linear regression analysis.

First, we conducted a multiple linear regression analysis with gray matter volume as dependent variable. Structural T1-weighted MRI scans were segmented into gray and white matter images after affine registration to the Montreal Neurological Institute (MNI) T1 template. Gray/white matter images were normalized and the deformation parameters were reapplied to the original whole-brain structural images. These images were segmented again and the gray matter images were multiplied by the Jacobian determinants derived from the spatial normalization step [182] [180]. The gray matter images were smoothed with a 12x12x12mm^3 full width of half maximum (FWHM) filter. The significance map of the regression analysis was thresholded at a voxel-level inference threshold of $P \prec 0.05$ corrected for the entire brain volume.

Second, we conducted a multiple linear regression analysis with brain response amplitude as dependent variable. EPI volumes were realigned and resliced using trilinear interpolation. A mean EPI volume was obtained during realignment and the structural MRI was co-registered with that mean volume. The structural scan was normalized to the MNI T1 template in Talairach space [182] [180] using non-linear basis functions. The same deformation parameters were applied to the EPI volumes which were subsequently spatially smoothed using a 6 mm FWHM isotropic Gaussian kernel. Data from different runs were proportionally scaled to a grand mean of 100 arbitrary units to account for overall differences in the intensity of whole brain volume across the time series. A high-pass filter of 216 sec was applied and a low-pass filter which consisted of a canonical hemodynamic response function (HRF). The epoch-related response was modeled by a canonical HRF, convolved with a boxcar. A t statistic for the parameter estimates was generated for each subject for the contrast between associative-semantic minus visuoperceptual conditions for words and pictures together and for the contrasts associative-semantic minus visuoperceptual condition for words or for pictures separately. The individuals' t maps were subsequently transformed to Z maps and entered into a second level analysis. At second level, we carried out a multiple linear regression analysis with fMRI response amplitude during associative-semantic versus visuoperceptual conditions as dependent variable and individual factor scores as regressors. The significance map was thresholded at a voxel-level inference threshold of $P \prec 0.05$ corrected for the entire brain volume.

In analogy with stroke recovery studies [198] [227], we calculated a laterality index: From the multiple linear regression group analysis, we selected the voxels of peak activation ($P \prec 0.05$ corrected) together with all brain voxels within a radius of 10 voxels from this peak, and for each voxel their contralateral counterpart. Within this bilateral volume of interest, we determined for each PPA subject and for each healthy control how many voxels were activated to the left and to the right during the associative-semantic versus the visuoperceptual condition at an uncorrected $P \prec 0.001$. Our laterality index (LI) was defined as: (L-R)/(L+R), with L the number of voxels activated to the left and R to the right.

2.4 Results

2.4.1 Neuropsychological data

	Factor 1	Factor 2	Factor 3	Factor 4
AAT				
Naming	**0.90**	0.19	0.04	-0.11
Comprehension	**0.88**	0.16	0.09	0.10
Token Test	-0.59	-0.17	-0.44	-0.34
Spontaneous speech	0.61	-0.2	0.49	0.12
PALPA	**0.87**	0.15	-0.04	0.01
Object Decision	0.67	0.47	-0.04	0.25
CPM	0.65	0.29	0.44	-0.07
TMT	-0.06	-0.12	**-0.82**	0.31
Number location	0.02	0.03	-0.11	**0.92**
AVLT				
Learning	0.43	0.68	0.35	0.12
Recall	0.24	**0.91**	0.09	0.03
% Recall	0.14	**0.90**	-0.03	-0.15
Recognition	0.13	0.78	0.14	0.15
RVDLT				
Recognition	-0.26	0.61	0.57	0.05

Table 2.4: Factor loadings: Correlation between the neuropsychological test scores and the factors that were extracted from the neuropsychological dataset by means of Factor Analysis. Bold: Factor loadings greater than 0.7. *Abbreviations:* See Table 2.2.

Factor analysis clustered the neuropsychological test scores of all 52 subjects by 4 factors; Table 2.4). Factor *1* explained 44.6% of the total variance (Eigenvalue: 6.7) and clustered the naming and comprehension tasks of the AAT and the PALPA verbal association task (Table 2.4). Factor *2* explained 16.4% of the total variance (Eigenvalue: 2.5) and clustered the delayed recall and recognition tasks of the Auditory Verbal Learning Test (AVLT). Factor *3* explained 10.1% of the total variance (Eigenvalue: 1.5) and consisted of the Trail Making Test B/A ratio [108]. The fourth factor (Factor *4*) correlated with the Number Location task [107], explaining 7.4% of the total variance (Eigenvalue: 1.1)).

	Reaction time (ms)			Accuracy (% correct)			Omissions		
	PPA	Controls	MCI	PPA	Controls	MCI	PPA	Controls	MCI
Semantic(P)	3551 (127)	3014 (100)	3077 (129)	67.8 (2.3)	81.0 (1.7)	78.8 (2.2)	15.6 (1.9)	6.2 (1.8)	5.8 (2.1[illegible]
Semantic(W)	3595 (130)	2866 (88)	2965 (113)	75.6 (2.9)	84.2 (2.0)	84.9 (1.9)	12.3 (2.0)	2.9 (1.8)	7.0 (2.2[illegible]
Visuoperc(P)	2969 (154)	2537 (94)	2702 (147)	80.6 (1.8)	88.9 (1.6)	87.7 (1.8)	6.5 (1.5)	3.3 (1.3)	5.6 (1.6[illegible]
Visuoperc(W)	2813 (117)	2355(88)	2400 (118)	84.4 (3.1)	90.1 (1.9)	88.1 (2.0)	6.3 (1.3)	2.0 (1.2)	4.7 (1.4[illegible]

Table 2.5: Reaction times, accuracies and omissions during the fMRI experiment (mean (s.e.)). *Abbreviations:* Semantic(P): Associative-semantic task with pictures; Semantic(W): Associative-semantic task with words; Visuoperc(P): Visuoperceptual task with pictures: Visuoperc(W): Visuoperceptual task with words.

Case	1	2	3	4	5	6	7	8	9	10	11	12	13	14	15	16	17	18	1[illegible]
Accuracy (% correct)																			
Semantic(P)	**64**	77	67	66	67	58	**63**	**53**	**56**	70	75	72	**54**	75	61	88	80	67	7[illegible]
Semantic(W)	72	75	87	68	75	69	81	**51**	**55**	74	90	80	**64**	88	**63**	92	88	73	9[illegible]
Visuoperc(P)	95	90	95	97	79	**65**	**73**	**61**	**64**	96	75	80	**69**	93	**59**	86	84	74	9[illegible]
Visuoperc(W)	95	96	97	98	84	68	**71**	**56**	**58**	98	82	91	79	100	**58**	96	100	80	9[illegible]
Reaction time (ms)																			
Semantic(P)	3773	3594	3735	3426	3560	2076	**4018**	3150	3644	3540	3531	2839	**4178**	3236	3830	3342	3870	**4044**	**409[illegible]**
Semantic(W)	**3985**	**4381**	**3787**	3572	3405	2110	**3665**	3101	3411	3585	3470	2877	**3899**	3577	**4154**	3359	**3763**	**4036**	**397[illegible]**
Visuoperc(P)	2658	2770	2989	2171	2978	1833	3204	2271	**3493**	2959	3154	2234	**3885**	2486	3071	2989	**3875**	**3877**	**352[illegible]**
Visuoperc(W)	2356	2513	2801	2286	2823	2054	**3243**	2190	**3432**	2802	3106	2448	2911	2316	**3592**	3004	2985	**3387**	**320[illegible]**

Table 2.6: Individual performance parameters during the fMRI experiment at time of inclusion. *Bold*: 2 standard deviations lower than average of our age- and education-matched healthy controls. Same conventions as in Table 2.5

2.4.2 Performance of the fMRI task

There was a main effect of group upon reaction times ($F(2,49)=7.1$, $P<0.01$), accuracies ($F(2,49)=5.1$, $P<0.01$) and omissions ($F(2,49)=5.2$, $P<0.01$) (Table 2.5 and Table 2.6). Post-hoc analysis revealed that PPA patients responded more slowly and less accurately than normals ($P<0.01$) and MCI patients ($P<0.05$) and made more omissions than normals ($P<0.01$).

There was a significant interaction between group and task ($F(2, 49)=6.2$, $P<0.01$): PPA patients made significantly more omissions during the semantic task relative to the visuoperceptual task than normals and MCI patients (Table 2.5 and Table 2.6). A similar trend was present for reaction times ($F(2, 49)=2.8$, $P=0.07$). There were no 3-way interactions between group, task and modality.

2.4.3 Neuroimaging results

Left anterior temporal *volume* correlated *positively* with individual scores on a cluster of language tests (factor *1*, Table 2.4): Left anterior temporal volume was smaller as individual language factor scores were lower (Fig. 2.1*D*). The correlation was significant both in lateral (-48,12,-24, Z=5.63, ext. 336, corr. $P\prec0.001$, r=0.67) and in medial anterior temporal cortex (-28,-6,-24, Z=4.93, ext. 295 , corr. $P\prec$ 0.05, r=0.63) (Fig. 2.1*C*).

The amplitude of *right* anterior temporal fMRI *responses* during the associative-semantic conditions compared to the visuoperceptual conditions correlated *inversely* with individual language factor scores (54,-3,-33, Z=4.77, ext. 35, corr. $P\prec0.05$, r=-0.62) (Fig. 2.1*A*,*B*): Right anterior temporal responses were stronger as individual language factor scores were lower (Fig. 2.1*B*). In the symmetrical left-sided anterior temporal cortex, the direction of the correlation was opposite: Response amplitude in left anterior temporal cortex was higher as individual language factor scores were better (-42,12,-24, Z=4.17, ext. 53, uncorr. $P\prec0.001$, r=0.53).

There was an effect of PPA subgroup upon brain volume and response: Left anterior temporal volume was significantly smaller in PPA patients with compared to those without word comprehension deficit (gray matter density: 0.37 (s.e. 0.06) and 0.56 (s.e. 0.02), respectively, $P\prec$ 0.005). Right anterior temporal response amplitude was higher in PPA patients with compared to those without word comprehension deficit (contrast-weighted sum of beta estimates 0.32 (s.e. 0.09) and -0.05 (s.e. 0.09), respectively, $P\prec0.05$).

The functional laterality index differed significantly between groups (PPA with comprehension deficit, PPA without comprehension deficit, MCI, normal controls) (one-way ANOVA, $F(3,48)=6.4$, $P\prec0.005$). According to a post-hoc analysis, the laterality index differed significantly between PPA with comprehension deficit and healthy controls ($P\prec0.0005$), between PPA without word comprehension deficit and healthy controls ($P\prec0.05$), between PPA with comprehension deficit and MCI ($P\prec0.005$), and between PPA with and without comprehension deficit ($P\prec0.05$). In the anterior temporal cortex of normal subjects, the activation during the associative semantic compared to the visuoperceptual task was more extensive in the left hemisphere (L=90.1 (s.e. 18.0); R=20.4 (s.e. 8.2); LI=0.64 (s.e. 0.11)) (Fig. 2.1*E*, *green*). Only in one normal control was the laterality index negative: This patient was left-handed (Fig. 2.1*E*). This left-sided preponderance was also true in the MCI group (L=82.7 (s.e. 20.6); R=38.5 (s.e. 12.5); LI=0.38 (s.e. 0.14)).

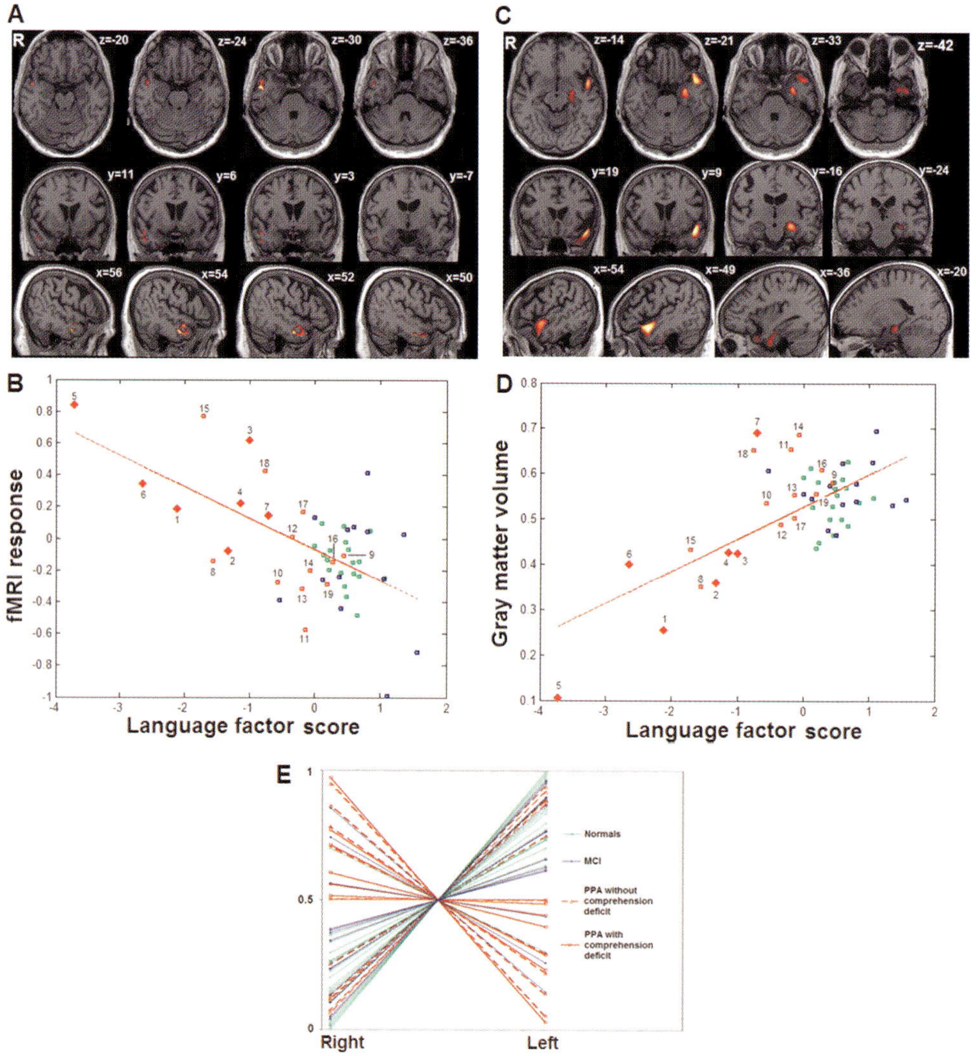

Figure 2.1: Multiple linear regression group analysis with individual factor scores as regressors. **A.** Multiple linear regression with fMRI response as dependent variable. Z map thresholded at $P < 0.05$ corrected for the total brain search volume. **B.** Regression plot. Each datapoint corresponds to one subject. X axis: Individual scores on the language factor (Factor 1, Table 2.4). Y axis: Amplitude of the fMRI response during associative semantic versus control conditions in the right anterior temporal cluster of significant activation. *Red:* PPA subjects. Numbers correspond to case indices in Table 2.2. *Red diamond*: PPA with comprehension deficit. *Red square*: PPA without comprehension deficit. *Green:* Normal controls. *Blue:* MCI controls. **C.** Multiple linear regression with gray matter volume as dependent variable. Z map thresholded at $P < 0.05$ corrected for the total brain search volume. **D.** Regression plot. X axis: Individual scores on the language factor (Factor 1). Y axis: Gray matter volume in the left anterior temporal cluster of significant activation. Same conventions as in *B*. **E.** Laterality index: Extent of left-sided versus right-sided activation (uncorrected $P < 0.001$) within the anterior temporal volume of interest for each individual. Each line corresponds to one subject. X axis: Left: Left anterior temporal half of the volume of interest, Right: Right anterior temporal half of the volume of interest. Y axis: Number of voxels activated either to the left or to the right for a given subject within the volume of interest, divided by the total number of voxels activated bilaterally. *Legend: Green*: Normal controls. *Red dashed line*: PPA without comprehension deficit. *Red solid line*: PPA with comprehension deficit. *Blue*: MCI.

Conversely, in PPA patients with word comprehension deficits, anterior temporal activation was more extensive to the right (L=14.8 (s.e. 29.6); R=28.9 (s.e. 13.4); LI=-0.34 (s.e. 0.19)) ((Fig. 2.1*E*) *red solid*). PPA patients without word comprehension deficits showed an intermediate pattern (L=61.4 (s.e. 22.7); R=35.7 (s.e. 22.7); LI=0.23 (s.e. 0.14)) (Fig. 2.1*E*) *red dashed*). The sum of activated voxels to the left and to the right did not differ significantly between groups (one-way ANOVA, $F(3,48)=0.81$, $P=0.49$).

In order to exclude differences in performance during the fMRI session as an explanation we conducted a multiple linear regression analysis with accuracies, reaction times or omissions during the fMRI tasks as regressors and fMRI response as dependent variable. This analysis did not yield any significant effects in left or right anterior temporal areas, even when the threshold was lowered to an uncorr. $P \prec 0.01$.

2.5 Discussion

In PPA right anterior temporal response amplitude increases as language abilities decrease (Fig. 2.1*A*, *B*). In the homotopical left-sided region, brain volume and responses decrease in parallel with language competence (Fig. 2.1*D*). In PPA with comprehension deficit in particular, anterior temporal activation during the associative-semantic compared to the visuoperceptual task was more extensive to the right than to the left, opposite to what is seen in normal controls (Fig. 2.1*E*). The laterality shift resulted from actual activity increases to the right in those patients who were most severely affected and was not exclusively caused by left-sided activity decreases (Fig. 2.1*B*).

Differences in fMRI task performance can be excluded as an explanation. The regressors of our analysis were derived from the neuropsychological assessment and not from performance during fMRI scanning. When we entered the performance parameters of the fMRI session into a regression analysis, the correlation remained far below significance. Furthermore, the relationship between language scores and fMRI response went in opposite directions in the two hemispheres. This cannot be attributed to aspecific task difficulty effects.

In aphasic stroke patients [199], a rightward shift of activation in the aphasic patients correlated inversely with picture naming performance [199] and was associated with poorer recovery than ipsilesional activity increases [199] [208]. This inverse relationship between right-hemispheric activity and language competence in stroke [207] [199] [208] is in accordance with the inverse relationship between right anterior temporal activity and language competence in PPA in our study (Fig. 2.1*B*).

Right anterior temporal hyperactivity may reflect compensatory mechanisms, failure to compensate, or changes in task-solving strategies. It may also be maladaptive: Transcallosal disinhibition [206] may result in right-sided activation that does not serve an actual semantic processing purpose. Historically, reports of cases of left-hemispheric stroke who suffered a subsequent right-hemispheric stroke and experienced worsening of aphasia have suggested an active role of the right hemisphere in language processing [228]. In classic studies of recovery after left-hemispheric stroke [229] [230] [231], lesion size correlated *positively* with recovery of comprehension and *inversely* with rates of improvement of word generation or sentence processing. These and other studies [232] [209] have led to the hypothesis that the right hemisphere can compensate for word comprehension but not for articulation or grammatical impairment. This lesion-based hypothesis fits with our observation in PPA that the anterior temporal laterality shift occurred primarily in those patients who had a comprehension deficit.

In aphasic stroke or tumor patients, active interference with right-hemispheric activity affects language performance [204] [212] [233] [211]. For instance, TMS above the right inferior frontal zone of hyper-activity increased response latency during a verb generation task [212]. Longitudinal interventional studies in PPA are required to determine the effect of similar manipulations upon language performance.

In neurodegenerative disease, such as PPA, recovery of function is unfortunately rare. Functional re-organisation nevertheless takes place under such conditions too [45] [234] [88] [85]. A recent fMRI study revealed activity increases outside the classic language network in non-fluent progressive aphasia [45]. Our findings differ form this previous report by the confinement of the activity increases to right-hemispheric areas homotopic to focal left-hemispheric areas of structural atrophy.

There was considerable variability between subjects (Fig. 2.1*B*, *D*, *E*). Decreased left-sided anterior temporal volume and increased right-sided anterior temporal activity were pronounced in PPA patients who had comprehension deficits compared with those who did not (Fig. 2.1*B* red diamonds versus red squares). This difference between the two subgroups is not caused by differences in overall disease severity: Syntactic production and articulation was *more* impaired in the PPA sample without word comprehension deficit than in the group with word comprehension deficit (Table 2.3). The double dissociation between word comprehension and articulatory and grammatical output is a classical feature of the clinical heterogeneity among PPA patients [6] [43] [7] [38] [235] [33] [236] [34]. Our data corroborate the view that this clinical heterogeneity reflects differences in underlying brain substrate.

Our left temporal findings confirmed previous volumetric [41] [44] [55] [237] and functional imaging studies [45] [55] in semantic dementia [44] [55] [237] and nonfluent progressive aphasia [44] [237]. Frontal changes were relatively weak compared with previous studies [44]. Our patients were on average less severely affected than those studied by Grossman and colleagues. Second, heterogeneity within the subgroup of PPA without comprehension deficit [38] [238] may also explain why frontal changes were relatively weak in our study.

Anterior temporal cortex is not a classical peri-sylvian language area. Until recently, herpes simplex encephalitis and surgical anterior temporal lobectomy were the principal neurological conditions that revealed how important anterior temporal integrity can be for language and semantic memory [21]. Detailed studies of cognition and anatomy in semantic dementia have drawn attention to the lateral and medial anterior temporal cortex as key structures for the processing of word meaning [32] [55] [41] [239]. Functional imaging studies of the intact brain have confirmed this view: Left anterior temporal cortex is activated during associative-semantic judgements compared with visuoperceptual judgements regardless of input modality, words, or pictures [5]. It is activated when subjects read stories compared with sequences of unconnected sentences [240] or sentences compared with random word sequences [241]. We propose that the left anterior temporal pole is an associative structure that binds together representations of meaning that are distributed over human cerebral cortex [241] [242] [18].

In conclusion, functional reorganization of the language system in PPA has several characteristics in common with aphasia in stroke or tumor patients: Activity shifts from the predominantly left-sided lesion site to the right, in particular, in those patients who have comprehension deficit. In the right hemisphere, activity correlates inversely with language performance. The anterior temporal laterality shift provides us with a brain measure for evaluating the effect of behavioral or drug interventions in PPA.

Chapter 3

Paradoxical features of word finding difficulty in primary progressive aphasia

Annals of Neurology, 57, 204-209, 2005
Rik Vandenberghe, MD, PhD,[1–3] Mathieu Vandenbulcke, MD,[3] Sandra Weintraub, PhD,[1] Nancy Johnson, PhD,[1] Kathleen Porke,[2] Cynthia K. Thompson, PhD,[1,4] and Marsel M. Mesulam, MD, [1]
From the [1]Cognitive Neurology and Alzheimer's Disease Center, Northwestern University Hospital Gasthuisberg; [2]Neurology Department, University Hospital Gasthuisberg, [3]Cognitive Neurology Laboratory Faculty of Medicine, Katholieke Universiteit Leuven, Belgium; and [4]Department of Communication Sciences and Disorders, Northwestern University, Evanston, IL.

3.1 Abstract

Impaired word retrieval is a main symptom of primary progressive aphasia (PPA). The cognitive features of its impairment in PPA are poorly understood. We studied 12 patients with PPA (6 English and 6 Dutch-speaking), 7 patients with early-stage clinically probable Alzheimer's disease (PRAD), 5 with mild cognitive impairment (MCI) and 15 age-matched cognitively intact controls. Subjects had to name a picture (the probe) which was preceded by a written word (the prime) that could be the correct name of the picture, a noun belonging to the same semantic subcategory (related prime), a semantically unrelated noun (unrelated prime), or a pseudoword (neutral control). Naming latencies were longer in PPA and PRAD than in controls. Critically, the interaction between group and prime type was highly significant. PPA patients named the probe more slowly following a related compared to an unrelated prime. In contrast, PRAD and MCI patients and normal controls tended to name the probe faster when preceded by a related prime. The semantic interference effect in PPA generalised across languages and PPA subtypes. We conclude that selection among competing word-forms sharing a same semantic field is abnormal in PPA. The semantic interference effect constitutes

	Identity	Sem. rel.	Sem. unrel.	Nonword
Primary Progressive Aphasia				
case 1	2226 (405)	5764 (853)	2446 (289)	3119 (477)
case 2	2285 (326)	4614 (643)	4373 (686)	3787 (498)
case 3	1882 (244)	2047 (327)	3054 (605)	2519 (459)
case 4	1487 (108)	2615 (448)	2167 (202)	2114 (162)
case 5	1457 (135)	1874 (154)	1945 (279)	2242 (481)
case 6	1572 (143)	3756 (531)	2631 (294)	2698 (338)
case 7	2222 (59)	2547 (80)	2500 (78)	2399 (85)
case 8	2092 (160)	3179 (261)	2538 (173)	2840 (230)
case 9	2340 (126)	3357 (240)	3091 (153)	3187(304)
case 10	1739 (59)	2516 (321)	2032 (110)	2289 (155)
case 11	2477 (197)	4857 (433)	3485 (301)	4139 (457)
case 12	2022 (198)	4170 (701)	3223 (589)	3940(474)
mean (s.e.)	**1981 (98)**	**3440 (216)**	**2790 (149)**	**2939 (144)**
Clinically probable Alzheimer's disease				
case 1	1977 (113)	3001 (200)	3129 (427)	2916 (373)
case 2	1746 (351)	1629 (58)	1797 (141)	1677 (102)
case 3	1333 (40)	1784 (125)	1785 (161)	1688 (120)
case 4	2038 (146)	2141 (95)	2480 (270)	2386 (260)
case 5	1755 (102)	2152 (135)	2024 (138)	2469 (325)
case 6	2378 (184)	2675 (220)	2877 (262)	2403 (165)
case 7	1694 (90)	2218 (209)	2282 (437)	1801 (66)
mean (s.e.)	**1845 (128)**	**2228 (283)**	**2339 (195)**	**2191 (189)**
Mild Cognitive Impairment				
mean (s.e.)	**1691 (152)**	**1942 (335)**	**1965 (231)**	**1938 (224)**
Cognitively Intact Controls				
mean (s.e.)	**1363 (87)**	**1489 (193)**	**1553 (133)**	**1533 (129)**

Table 3.2: Reaction times in ms in the 4 types of priming trials (mean and standard deviation (between brackets)) and the 4 subject groups. Cases 1 to 6: English-speaking PPA patients, cases 7 to 12: Dutch-speaking PPA patients. Cases 1,2,3,7,8,9,10: Non-fluent PPA, cases 4,5,6,11,12: Fluent PPA.

Critically, the interaction between group and prime type was significant ($F(9,105)$ 7.4, $P \prec 0.00001$) (Fig. 3.1*A*). According to planned comparisons, the reaction time difference between semantically related and unrelated primes differed significantly between PPA patients and normals ($F(1,35)$ 9.7, $P \prec 0.005$), between PPA and PRAD ($F(1,35)$ 7.4, $P \prec 0.05$) and between PPA and MCI ($F(1,35)$ 4.6, $P \prec 0.05$) (Fig. 3.1*A*): PPA patients were significantly slower following a semantically related prime in comparison to a semantically unrelated prime ($P \prec 0.000005$) (Table 3.2, Fig. 3.1*A*), in contrast with cognitively intact controls, patients with PRAD and patients with MCI. During semantically related priming trials reaction times were significantly longer in PPA than in PRAD ($P \prec 0.02$), MCI ($P \prec 0.01$) or cognitively intact controls ($P \prec 0.00001$) while reaction times during the semantically unrelated priming trials did not differ significantly between the PPA versus PRAD or MCI patients ($P \succ 0.1$).

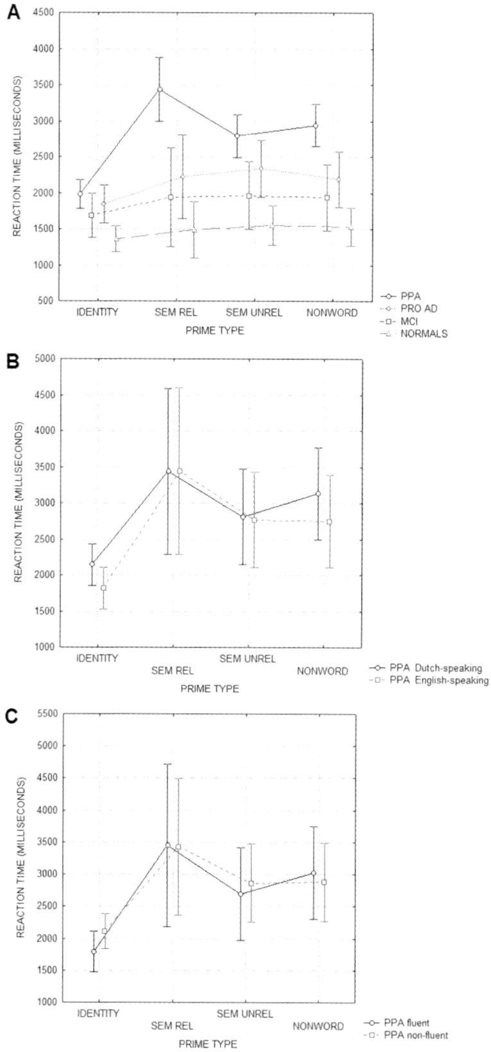

Figure 3.1: Primed picture naming. Reaction times (mean and s.e.) plotted as a function of prime type. **A.** PPA patients were significantly slower following a semantically related prime in comparison to a semantically unrelated prime. The cognitively intact controls and the patients with PRAD and MCI tended to be faster following a semantically related prime in comparison to a semantically unrelated prime. *Legend:* Blue solid line: PPA; Red dotted line: PRAD; Magenta triangles: MCI; Green diamonds: Normal controls. **B,C.** PPA subgroup analysis. *B.* Effect of language. Dark blue solid line: Dutch-speaking; Cyan dashed line: English-speaking. *C.* Effect of fluency. Dark blue solid line: Fluent PPA; Cyan dashed line: Non-fluent PPA patients. *Abbreviations:* Sem rel: Semantically related; Sem unrel: Semantically unrelated; PPA: Primary progressive aphasia; PRAD: Clinically probable Alzheimer's disease; MCI: Mild cognitive impairment.

We performed two subgroup analyses. First, we performed a repeated-measures ANOVA with group as between-subjects factor (2 levels: Dutch- versus English-speaking PPA) and prime type as within-subjects factor (4 levels: Identity, semantically related, semantically unrelated and pseudoword) (Fig. 3.1*B*). As Fig. 3.1*B* indicates, Dutch speaking and English speaking PPA patients showed the same semantic interference effect (F(3,30) 0.37, p≻0.7). This also implicates that the findings are independent of the two different ways in which responses were recorded (manual versus digital). Second, we performed a repeated-measures ANOVA with group (2 levels: Fluent and non-fluent PPA) and prime type (Fig. 3.1*C*). As Fig. 3.1*C* indicates, fluent and non-fluent PPA patients showed the same semantic interference effect (F(3,30) 0.39, p≻0.7).

There was no correlation between the priming effect and disease duration.

In PPA the total number of errors was also influenced by the type of prime. PPA subjects made significantly more errors following a semantically related (32%, s.e. 7) compared to a semantically unrelated prime (27%, s.e. 6.9) (Student's paired t 2.6 (d.f. 11), P≺0.05). The proportion of errors consisting of a repetition of the prime or of the first syllable of the prime was also significantly larger following a semantically related prime (21.7%, s.e. 7.1) in comparison to a semantically unrelated prime (1.5%, s.e. 1.0) (Student's paired t 2.77 (d.f. 5), P≺0.05). In MCI and PRAD, the total number of errors was approximately equal following semantically related (15.2%, s.e. 2.8) and unrelated primes (15.9%, s.e. 3.4) (Student's paired t 0.5 (d.f. 11)).

3.5 Discussion

In PPA, word retrieval was significantly slower and more error-prone following a semantically related prime than a semantically unrelated prime (Table 3.2; Fig. 3.1*A*). This paradoxical negative priming effect generalised across different languages (Fig. 3.1*B*) and PPA subtypes (Fig. 3.1*C*). It was highly consistent among subjects despite heterogeneity in disease duration and the wide range of severity of anomia (Table 3.2). A different pattern of priming was obtained in PRAD, MCI and normal controls who showed faster word retrieval in response to a semantically related prime (Table 3.2; Fig. 3.1*A*). The difference between PPA and PRAD indicates that the semantic interference pattern is not a non-specific consequence of "general cognitive loss".

The facilitatory priming by semantically related items in normal controls is expected given the long stimulus onset asynchrony [165] and the fact that we did not explicitly exclude semantically related primes with a high degree of associative linkage to the probe [166]. The preservation or augmentation of this semantic priming in early-stage PRAD also replicates previous findings [251] [252] [253] (Table 3.2).

Our findings in PPA differ from a semantic priming study of auditory lexical decision in a single case of semantic dementia [260] in whom semantic priming did not differ from that found in normal controls. Two of our patients, cases 11 and 12, fulfilled the criteria for semantic dementia [7], yet showed a strong interference effect. One possible explanation is the SOA difference between the two studies (200-250 ms [260] versus 750 ms in our study). Further studies are required to examine the effect of parametric variations of SOA or proportion of different prime types to tease apart reflexive and cognitive components [261] [262] in different PPA subgroups.

Semantic interference has been described in neurological patients before. In Broca aphasics, "inhibitory semantic priming" was found in a lexical decision task when the list contained a high proportion of semantically related primes. An analogous process of "retrieval inhibition" has also been described in a picture naming task in anomic temporal lobe epilepsy subjects [263].

The pathological interference seen in PPA can be understood in analogy with models for attentional search [264] [265]. The Theory of Visual Attention [264] [265] offers a mathematical account of why subjects spend more effort searching for a target within a stimulus array as the similarity between the target and the distractors increases. It explains patterns of attentional search in terms of discriminability and behavioral pertinence [264] [265]. We postulate that PPA interferes with the discriminability of semantically related word forms during lexical retrieval even at stages when semantic processing is relatively spared. According to this scenario, the prime activates the proper semantic field and paradoxically slows the naming of semantically related probes because the correct choice becomes embedded in a field of semantically related lexical items with similar activity levels. Impaired selection among word-forms that are connected to the same semantic field can be due to degradation of a semantic field [113] [32], to changes in the connections of the semantic field with word-form networks [147] or to changes within the word form networks themselves [147] [266] [267]. The actual locus of impairment may vary among PPA patients [267].

To conclude, naming is impaired in PPA due to alteration of the process of selecting among competing word codes belonging to the same semantic field [147]. This selection deficit generalises across language groups and PPA subtypes and disease stages and constitutes a positive feature distinguishing PPA from PRAD and MCI.

Chapter 4

Progression of anomia in primary progressive aphasia: Neural predictors and correlates

Paper in preparation
Mathieu Vandenbulcke[1,2], Natalie Nelissen[1], Katrien Fannes[1], Kathleen Porke[4], Ronald Peeters[3], Rik Vandenberghe[1,4]
[1]Cognitive Neurology Laboratory, Section Experimental Neurology, K.U. Leuven, [2]Psychiatry Department, [3]Radiology Department, [4]Neurology Department, University Hospital Gasthuisberg, Leuven, Belgium

4.1 Abstract

In this longitudinal study, we identified neural predictors and correlates of naming decline in PPA. Eighteen PPA patients and 15 healthy subjects participated. Subjects underwent neuropsychological assessment, structural and functional magnetic resonance imaging (MRI) at time of inclusion and after one year of follow-up. To identify neural predictors of naming decline, we compared gray matter volume at time of inclusion between patients who declined over a one-year period and patients who did not. To study the neural substrate of progression of naming impairment, we correlated change of naming performance with change of gray matter volume. A higher degree of left anterior temporal atrophy was associated with a faster rate of naming decline. Naming decline correlated with progressive left posterior inferior temporal and right-sided temporal atrophy. Longitudinal structural MRI provides us with a brain measure that is sensitive to cognitive change and may be used to monitor treatment effects in PPA.

4.2 Introduction

Anomia is a key diagnostic feature of primary progressive aphasia [43] and the neural substrate of picture naming impairment has been well-documented in cross-sectional studies of PPA [41] [44] [174] [175]. To our knowledge, none of the longitudinal studies of PPA [268] [269] [270] [271] [34] [272] [211] has quantified cortical gray matter changes associated with progression of picture naming impairment so far. We examined the sensitivity of longitudinal structural MRI, using voxel-based morphometry (VBM) [184] [185] [186] [273] [187], to predict and detect language decline in PPA.

Longitudinal neuroimaging studies of memory decline in Alzheimer's disease (AD) may provide us with clues about the neural substrate of language decline in PPA. In mild cognitive impairment (MCI) and Alzheimer's disease (AD), the degree of hippocampal and entorhinal atrophy is predictive of memory decline [274] [275]. Medial temporal atrophy also predicts conversion from MCI to AD [187] [276] [277] [275] [278] [63]. In probable Alzheimer's Disease (AD), progression of gray matter volume loss is a measure of disease progression [279] [275] [280] [273] [281] [282] [283] [284] [187] [274] and is currently tested as a surrogate marker to monitor treatment effects.

Based on the findings in AD, we made the following predictions in PPA: First, we hypothesized that the main areas of gray matter loss associated with naming impairment cross-sectionally would also be predictive of naming decline within one year of follow-up. These areas include the left anterior temporal [41] [44] [174] [175] and left prefrontal cortex [44]. Second, we predicted that the neural substrate of progression of naming impairment would extend beyond the areas that correlate with naming impairment cross-sectionally.

4.3 Subjects and Methods

4.3.1 Subjects

A cohort of eighteen patients who fulfilled the criteria for primary progressive aphasia (PPA) [6] [43] participated, 10 men and 8 women, between 45 and 78 years of age (mean 67.1, s.d. 8.9 years), with a mean educational level of 12.5 years (s.d. 2.9) and a mean Oldfield score of +90.3 [225]. One PPA subject was left-handed (Oldfield score -73). Word retrieval problems were the primary reason for attending the memory clinic in all patients. Neuropsychological examination confirmed language impairment in all PPA subjects with relative sparing of other cognitive domains at time of inclusion (for details, see Vandenbulcke et al. [174]). Six of the 18 PPA patients (cases 2, 3, 5, 5, 12, and 17) had a significant single word comprehension deficit and object agnosia during initial evaluation [174] and fulfilled the criteria for semantic dementia according to the Lund-Manchester criteria [7] (Table 4.1).

A healthy control cohort consisted of 15 normal subjects, matched for gender (9 men, 6 women), age (mean age 65.6, s.d. 4.1), educational level (12.4 years, s.d. 2.6), and handedness (Oldfield score +90.8) [225]. As in the PPA group, 1 control subject was left-handed (Oldfield score -64).

The 19 PPA patients and 15 healthy controls underwent neuropsychological assessment, functional and structural MRI at time of inclusion and after one year of follow-up. Mean

ase	1	2	3	4	5	6	7	8	9	10	11	12	13	14	15	16	17	18
ge	45	70	64	51	59	76	65	74	68	57	74	69	66	71	78	72	74	77
ducation	12	6	10	15	12	17	14	15	12	20	14	14	12	12	12	12	8	12
isease duration	2	7	2	2	5	2	2	3	4	5	4	2	3	5	2	12	2	4
AT																		
Naming																		
t0	**-7.97**	**-9.90**	**-9.66**	**-12.8**	**-10.4**	**-4.73**	**-3.41**	-0.04	-1.24	**-1.97**	**-8.45**	**-7.49**	-0.04	**-4.37**	-0.28	-0.76	**-2.21**	**-3.41**
Δt	**-27.6**	**-6.24**	**-5.56**	**-5.22**	**-4.21**	**-3.87**	-1.84	-1.84	-1.50	-0.83	-0.48	-0.15	0.18	0.86	1.20	1.54	1.54	3.57
Word comp																		
Auditory																		
t0	**-3.48**	**-2.95**	**-6.09**	**-8.18**	**-8.18**	**-2.43**	-0.34	-0.87	-5.04	0.69	**-3.48**	**-2.43**	**-3.48**	-0.34	**-2.43**	**-2.43**	**-4.52**	**-4.00**
Δt	-0.83	**-3.13**	0.32	0.03	0.60	**-0.83**	-0.25	0.31	0.60	0.31	1.18	0.89	0.60	0.32	1.46	0.89	1.75	1.46
Visual																		
t0	-0.74	**-6.26**	**-6.28**	**-17.37**	-17.37	-1.66	0.18	-0.74	**-3.51**	1.10	-1.66	**-2.58**	**-7.20**	-1.66	1.11	-1.66	-4.43	1.11
Δt	**-5.44**	-0.54	**-2.17**	2.72	3.13	-0.54	-0.13	1.08	0.27	0.27	-0.14	1.90	3.13	1.08	0.27	0.68	1.08	-1.36
Total																		
t0	**-2.82**	**-4.71**	**-6.98**	**-13.04**	**-13.04**	**-2.45**	-0.17	-0.93	**-5.09**	0.95	**-3.20**	**-2.82**	**-5.47**	-0.93	-1.31	**-2.45**	-5.09	**-2.45**
Δt	**-3.73**	**-2.85**	-1.09	1.32	1.98	-1.09	-0.44	0.65	0.44	0.22	0.66	1.54	1.97	0.87	1.09	0.65	1.75	0.22
Repetition																		
t0	**-8.15**	**-3.78**	0.58	0.58	0.58	-1.60	**-16.9**	-1.60	0.58	**-40.9**	**-25.6**	**-3.78**	0.58	**-8.15**	**-5.97**	**-14.7**	0.58	0.58
Δt	**-118**	**-4.51**	**-4.58**	**-2.33**	-0.14	-0.14	**-32.9**	**-4.51**	**-6.69**	**-19.8**	**-35.0**	**-4.51**	**-8.88**	-0.14	4.22	4.22	**-2.33**	**-6.69**
Token Test																		
t0	-0.66	**4.78**	0.24	**6.60**	**8.42**	**9.33**	**15.7**	-0.66	0.24	**13.9**	**5.69**	1.15	**8.42**	**2.06**	**7.51**	0.24	**2.97**	**7.51**
Δt	**-9.10**	-1.43	**4.31**	**6.23**	-0.47	**4.31**	-0.48	-0.47	0.47	**13.9**	**11.0**	-1.43	**-4.32**	**2.39**	-7.19	-0.47	-1.43	**17.7**
ALPA																		
t0	**-3.73**	**-5.27**	**-3.73**	**-9.11**	**-5.27**	**-2.96**	0.10	-0.66	**-2.20**	0.10	**-2.20**	**-6.04**	-1.43	0.10	**-2.20**	**-2.20**	**-5.27**	**-2.96**
Δt	**-5.63**	0.12	**-3.90**	**-5.63**	**-3.33**	1.28	**-2.17**	0.70	-0.44	0.70	1.28	1.28	-1.60	-1.60	-1.02	1.28	2.43	0.70
bject decision																		
t0	**-2.43**	-1.88	**-2.99**	**-3.54**	**-5.76**	**-2.99**	**-2.99**	2.54	**-2.99**	1.44	-1.32	-0.22	**-2.43**	-0.22	-1.88	-0.77	**-4.10**	**-3.54**
Δt	2.15	0.55	0.15	-0.24	-1.44	2.55	3.35	-1.44	0.95	-0.24	1.35	0.55	1.35	0.55	-0.24	2.15	2.55	1.75

Table 4.1: Z-scores of language test performance. *t0*: Z-score of performance at time of inclusion. Δt: Z-score of change of performance within one year of follow-up. *Bold:* Z-score below -1.96 (or above 1.96 in case of Token Test). Age and education in years. Case indices correspond to the numbers in Fig. 4.2, Fig. 4.1 and Fig. 4.3. *Abbreviations:* AAT: Aachen Aphasie Test. Word comp: Word comprehension. PALPA: Psycholinguistic Assessment of Language Processing in Aphasia. Mean score and SD of test performance of controls used for calculation of Z-scores at time of inclusion: AAT naming: 117.2 (SD 4.16), AAT auditory single word comprehension: 28.7 (SD 1.91), Visual single word comprehension: 28.8(SD 1.08), AAT comprehension total: 57.5 (SD 2.64), AAT repetition: 149.4 (SD 0.91), Token Test: 0.73 (SD 1.09), PALPA verbal association: 28.9 (SD 1.30), BORB object decision: 27.4 (SD 1.80) Mean change and SD of test scores of controls used for calculation of Z-scores of change: AAT naming: 0.44 (SD 2.95), AAT auditory single word comprehension: -1.11 (SD 3.47), Visual single word comprehension: -0.66 (SD 2.44), AAT comprehension total: -1.0 (SD 4.55), AAT repetition: 0.06 (SD 0.45), Token Test: 0.5 (SD 1.04), PALPA verbal association: -0.22 (SD 1.73), BORB object decision: -2.38 (SD 2.55)

interval between baseline and follow-up assessment was 13.4 months (s.d. 1.7) (range between 12 and 17 months) in PPA and 14.7 months (s.d. 2.3) (range between 12 and 19 months) in controls.

All subjects gave written informed consent in accordance with the Declaration of Helsinki. The study protocol was approved by the Ethical Committee, University Hospital Gasthuisberg, Leuven.

4.3.2 Language assessment and analysis

Our neurolinguistic battery was comprised of the Dutch version of the Aachen Aphasie Test, ("Akense Afasie Test", AAT)[101], the verbal associative-semantic task of the validated Dutch version of the Psycholinguistic Assessment of Language Processing in Aphasia (PALPA)[102]

[103] and the object decision test of the Birmingham Object Recognition Battery (BORB) [106].

The naming scores were derived from the naming test of the AAT, which includes picture naming of objects, colors and actions. To determine naming decline, we calculated for each subject a Z-score of change in naming performance based on the mean change and SD of controls. Significant progression was defined by a Z score below -1.96. Patients with significant progression of naming performance were classified as decliners, others as non-decliners.

We also calculated Z scores of changes for the other language tasks: The single word comprehension test (AAT), consisting of auditory and visual word-picture matching, the verbal associative-semantic task (PALPA), the single word repetition test (AAT), consisting of one-syllable, multi-syllable and morphologically complex words, the token test and the object decision task of the BORB. We also transformed language test scores at time of inclusion and at follow-up into Z-scores.

4.3.3 Voxel-based morphometry experiment

A 1.5 tesla Siemens Sonata system (Siemens Medical Solutions, Erlangen, Germany) equipped with an 8-channel receive-only head coil (MRI Devices Corp., Waukesha, USA) provided a T1-weighted structural volume (coronal inversion recovery prepared three-dimensional gradient echo images (MPRAGE); Inversion time 800 ms, TE/TR 3.93/1950 ms, flip angle 12, 1 mm isotropic in-plane resolution).

We used optimized voxel-based morphometry for the analysis of gray matter volume [184] [185] [186]. We first created a T1-template based upon 34 elderly controls (mean age: 67.4 y, SD 7.9y) [185]: We registered the 34 T1-weighted images onto the MNI T1 template using linear transformation functions (affine normalization), generated a mean image and smoothed with an 8 mm FWHM Gaussian kernel. The affine normalized whole brain images were segmented using the SPM99 algorithm and the resulting gray matter, white matter and cerebrospinal fluid (CSF) maps were averaged across all 34 controls to obtain custom prior probability images (i.e. a gray matter, white matter and CSF map). The optimized VBM protocol, applied to the MR images of the 18 PPA patients and 15 controls, consisted of affine registration to our T1 template followed by segmentation of the structural T1-weighted MRI scans into gray and white matter images. Gray matter images were normalized to our gray matter template using non-linear iterations and the deformation parameters were reapplied to the original whole-brain T1-weighted MRI images. These images were segmented again and the gray matter images were multiplied by the Jacobian determinants derived from the spatial normalization step. The gray matter images were smoothed with a 12x12x12mm^3 full width of half maximum (FWHM) filter. Gray matter volume changes within one year were quantified by subtracting the gray matter volume images obtained during initial and follow-up scanning. The resulting images contain the gray matter volume change on a voxel-by-voxel basis.

To identify structural predictors of naming decline, we compared gray matter volume of decliners with gray matter volume of non-decliners at time of inclusion using a two-sample t test. We extracted gray matter volumes from areas that significantly differed between decliners and non-decliners and entered these volumes together with initial naming scores as regressors in a stepwise multiple regression analysis with change of naming score as dependent variable.

To correlate naming decline with changes of gray matter volume, we conducted a linear regression analysis (SPM02) with Z-scores of change in naming performance entered as regressors and gray matter volume change as dependent variable. All significance maps were thresholded at a voxel level inference threshold of $P \prec 0.001$ and a cluster level threshold of $P \prec 0.05$ corrected for multiple comparisons in the entire brain volume.

4.3.4 fMRI experiment

We used the fMRI experiment to determine the functional significance of the structural predictors and correlates of naming decline. The design and acquisition protocol of the fMRI experiment has been described elsewhere [174] [285] [286]. In brief, the design was factorial. The first factor, task, had two levels: Associative-semantic versus visuoperceptual judgment. The second factor, input modality, also had two levels: Pictures versus printed words. Subjects had to press a left- or right-hand key depending on which of the two test stimuli matched the sample stimulus more closely in meaning or in size. We acquired T2* echo-planar images (EPI) (TE/TR 40/3000 ms, 42 sagittal slices, voxel size 3x3x3 mm^3) [174] [285] [286]. EPI volumes were processed using SPM02. A *t* statistic for the parameter estimates was generated for each subject for the contrast between associative-semantic minus visuoperceptual conditions for words and pictures together. The individuals' *t* maps were subsequently transformed to *Z* maps and entered in random-effects analysis.

Using a one-sample *t* test, we determined where the associative semantic conditions yielded higher activity than the visuoperceptual conditions at time of inclusion across subjects (thresholded at a voxel-level inference threshold of $P \prec 0.001$ and a cluster-level threshold of $P \prec 0.05$ corrected for the entire brain volume). We determined the overlap between the associative semantic system across subjects and the areas that were predictive of or correlated with naming decline. We extracted the fMRI response from the overlapping areas and compared the fMRI response between controls and PPA (corrected $P \prec 0.05$).

4.4 Results

4.4.1 Neuropsychological data

Significant progression of naming impairment was present in 6 patients (cases 1 to 6). These patients were classified as decliners. 4 out of six patients with naming decline also deteriorated on the verbal association task of the PALPA (cases 1, 3, 4 and 5), 2 on single word comprehension of the AAT (case 1 and 2), 4 on the token test (1 to 4), 4 on the single word repetition task (cases 1 to 4) and none on the object decision task (Table 4.1). Disease duration did not differ between decliners and non-decliners (3.3 years and 3.9 years respectively, Students t test $= -0.45$; $p = 0.7$) The change of naming score of case 1 was an extreme outlier according to an outlier detection analysis (STATISTICA version 6, StatSoft, Inc, OK, U.S) and was excluded for the correlation analyses.

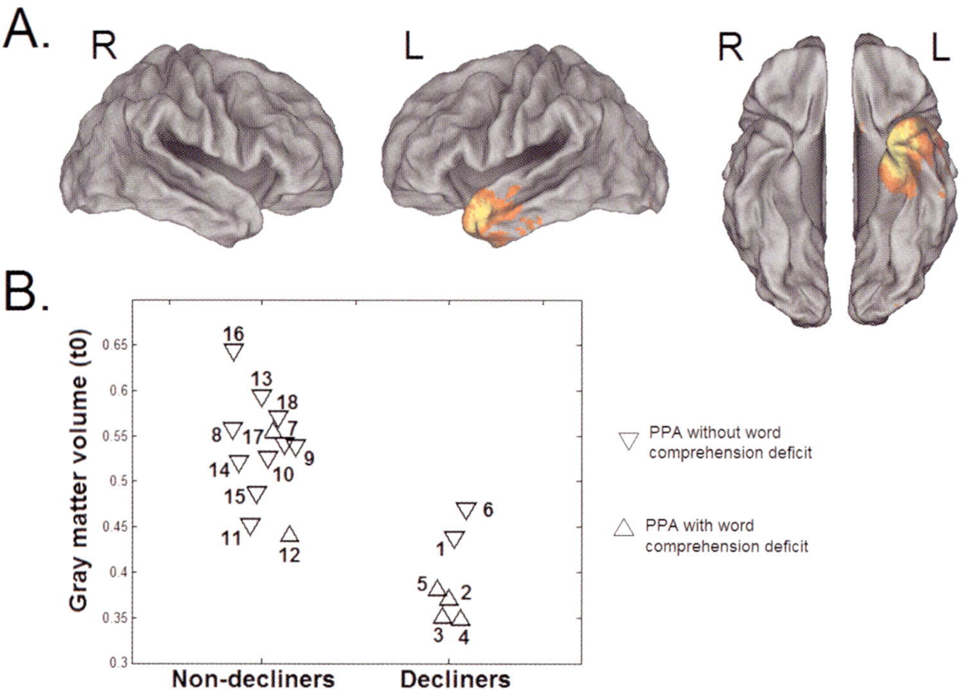

Figure 4.1: Predictors of progression of anomia. **A** Significance map of correlation between gray matter volume at time of inclusion and change of AAT naming score. Threshold: Uncorrected $P \prec 0.001$. Significance maps are superposed onto the template brain using CARET software (Washington University School of Medicine, Department of Anatomy and Neurobiology, http://brainmap.wustl.edu)**B** Plot of gray matter volume of the anterior temporal cluster depicted in **A**. Upward triangles: PPA with single word comprehension deficit, downward triangles: PPA without single word comprehension deficit, circles: Controls.

4.4.2 Neuroimaging results

Structural imaging results

Left anterior temporal lobe atrophy at time of inclusion was predictive of naming decline: Gray matter volume of the left anterior temporal lobe was significantly lower in patients who declined on picture naming over the next year compared to patients who did not (-30,-4,-46, Z=4.04, ext. 2398, corr. $P \prec 0.001$) (Fig. 4.1). The four patients with the lowest anterior temporal volumes (cases 2, 3, 4, and 5) (Fig. 4.1) also had significant single word comprehension impairment at time of inclusion. A stepwise multiple regression analysis revealed that, in contrast with initial naming score (P = 0.6), anterior temporal volume ($P \prec 0.05$), was an independent predictor of naming decline.

Change of naming performance correlated significantly with gray matter volume loss of the left posterior inferior temporal gyrus (-48,-44,-22, Z=4.11, ext. 535, corr. $P \prec 0.001$, r= 0.81).

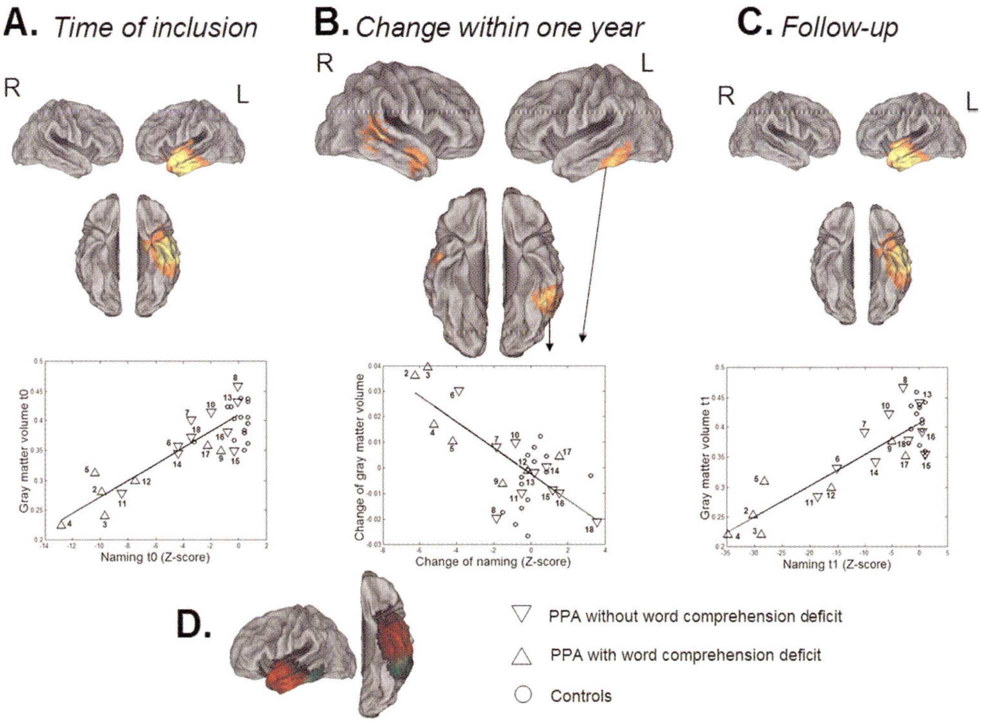

Figure 4.2: Cross-sectional and longitudinal correlations between naming and gray matter volume. **A** Correlation between AAT naming score and gray matter volume at time of inclusion (-46, 10,-12, Z=5.54, ext. 9587, corr. $P<0.001$, r= 0.88). **B** Correlation between change of AAT naming score and change of gray matter volume between time of inclusion and follow-up. **C** Correlation between AAT naming score and gray matter volume at follow-up (-44, 10, -12, Z=5.26, ext. 8903, corr. $P<0.001$, r= 0.86). **D** Comparison of the results of **a,** ***red*** and **b,** ***green***. Same conventions as Figure 4.1. Threshold: Uncorrected $P<0.001$.

In the right hemisphere, naming decline correlated with gray matter volume changes of the anterior (56,4,-30, Z=3.76, ext. 186, corr. $P<0.05$, r= 0.76) and posterior (56,-34,0, Z=4.38, ext. 758, corr. $P<0.001$, r= 0.83) middle temporal gyrus (Fig. 4.2 *B*). Gray matter volume change of the left posterior inferior temporal cluster (Fig. 4.2 *B*) also correlated significantly with change of single word comprehension (AAT) performance (r=0.68, $P<0.05$). The correlation between gray matter volume decrease and the change of naming (r= 0.81) was significantly higher than the correlation with change of repetition (r=-0.08), token test (r=0.07) and object decision (r=-0.02) ($P<0.05$). Gray matter volume of the left posterior inferior temporal gyrus decreased significantly more in patients with single comprehension deficit at time of inclusion compared with patients without ($P<0.05$).

Functional imaging results

The left posterior inferior temporal cluster described above (Fig. 4.2 *B*) overlapped with the system activated during associative semantic judgements with words and pictures across subjects (Fig. 4.3 *B*) (-48,-51,-21, Z=4.32, ext. 40, corr. $P \prec 0.001$). Functional MRI response in this overlapping area (Fig. 4.3 *B*) was significantly lower in PPA than in controls ($P \prec 0.05$). Without case 14, fMRI response in left inferotemporal cortex was not significantly lower in PPA compared to controls (P=0.065). Separate group analyses revealed that posterior temporal cortex was activated during the associative-semantic conditions relative to the visuoperceptual conditions in controls (corr. $P \prec 0.05$)(Fig. 4.3 *A*: *left*) but not in PPA (Fig. 4.3 *A*: *right*) (uncorr. $P \succ 0.001$). As shown in (Fig. 4.2 *B*), there was no difference in left inferotemporal fMRI response between patients who declined (cases 1 to 6) on the naming task compared to patients who did not (case 9 to 19).

Performances of the fMRI task are shown in Table 4.2 and Table 4.3. PPA patients were slower (F(1,31)=22.4, $P \prec 0.00005$), less accurate (F(1,31)=11.0, $P \prec 0.0005$) and made more omissions (F(1,31)=8.7, $P \prec 0.01$) than normals. There was a significant interaction between group and task: PPA patients made significantly more omissions during the semantic task relative to the visuoperceptual task than normals (F(1,31)=14.2, $P \prec 0.001$)

	Reaction time (ms)		Accuracy (% correct)		Omissions	
	PPA	controls	PPA	controls	PPA	controls
Semantic(P)						
t0	3584 (100)	2923 (111)	67.8 (2.1)	81.4 (2.2)	15.2 (2.2)	6.0 (2.3)
t1	3574 (127)	2800 (140)	70.5 (2.4)	82.0 (2.3)	28.9 (4.7)	9.2 (5.1)
Semantic(W)						
t0	3616 (92)	2809 (101)	75.5 (2.6)	84.8 (2.2)	12.1 (2.0)	2.7 (2.1)
t1	3625 (122)	2660 (129)	75.4 (3.1)	87.4 (2.9)	32.1 (4.7)	7.4 (5.2)
Visuoperc(P)						
t0	2948 (127)	2417 (141)	82.3 (2.5)	90.2 (2.7)	5.7 (1.3)	3.4 (1.4)
t1	2880 (126)	2272 (139)	79.4 (3.1)	91.7 (3.2)	21.2 (5.2)	7.0 (5.6)
Visuoperc(W)						
t0	2780 (108)	2218 (119)	86.1 (2.9)	91.9 (2.4)	5.5 (1.2)	1.9 (1.3)
t1	2733 (126)	2087 (139)	84.8 (3.2)	93.6 (3.3)	18.6 (5.1)	6.6 (5.5)

Table 4.2: Reaction times, accuracies and omissions during the fMRI experiment (mean (s.e.)). *Abbreviations:* T0: Initial scan; t1: follow-up scan; Semantic(P): Associative-semantic task with pictures; Semantic(W): Associative-semantic task with words; Visuoperc(P): Visuoperceptual task with pictures: Visuoperc(W): Visuoperceptual task with words.

Case	1	2	3	4	5	6	7	8	9	10	11	12	13	14	15	16	17	1
Accuracy (% correct)																		
Semantic(P)	**53**	66	77	**57**	**64**	80	70	88	72	**56**	**61**	67	75	**54**	76	75	**63**	6
Semantic(W)	**51**	68	75	67	72	88	74	92	80	**55**	**63**	87	90	**64**	91	88	81	7
Visuoperceptual(P)	**61**	97	89	96	95	84	96	86	80	**64**	**59**	95	**75**	**69**	96	93	**73**	**7**
Visuoperceptual(W)	**56**	98	96	97	95	100	98	96	91	**58**	**58**	97	82	79	97	100	**71**	8
Reaction time (ms)																		
Semantic(P)	3150	3426	3594	3536	3773	**3870**	2680	3342	2839	3644	**3830**	3735	3531	**4178**	**4095**	3236	**4018**	**404**
Semantic(W)	3101	**3572**	**4381**	3380	**3985**	**3763**	2703	3359	2877	3411	**4154**	**3787**	**3470**	**3899**	**3979**	**3577**	**3665**	**403**
Visuoperceptual(P)	2271	2171	2770	2206	2658	**3875**	2215	2989	2234	**3493**	3071	2989	3154	**3885**	**3521**	2486	3204	**387**
Visuoperceptual(W)	2190	2286	2513	2164	2356	2985	2108	3004	2448	**3432**	**3592**	2801	**3106**	2911	**3200**	2316	**3243**	**338**

Table 4.3: Individual performance parameters during the fMRI experiment at time of inclusion. *Bold*: 2 standard deviations lower than average of our age- and education-matched controls. Same conventions as in Table 4.2

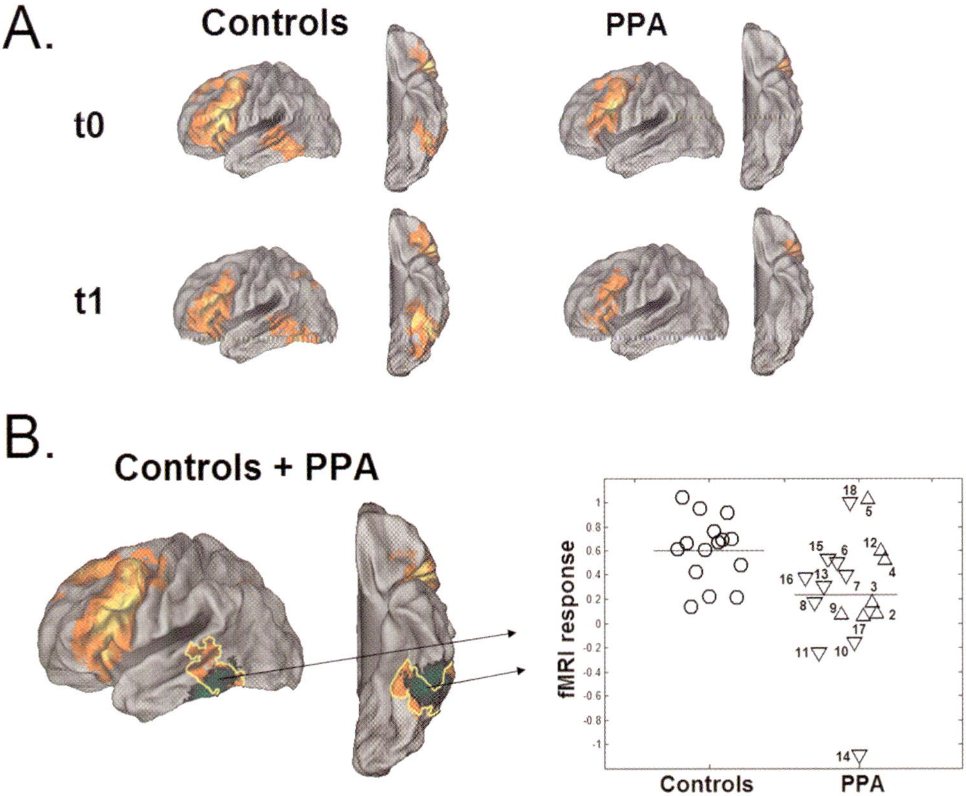

Figure 4.3: Posterior temporal fMRI response in PPA and controls **A** Significance maps from the subtraction associative-semantic minus visuoperceptual conditions in controls (*left*) and PPA (*right*) at time of inclusion (*upper*) and at follow-up (*lower*). **B** Plot of fMRI response from overlap between significance map (yellow) from the substraction associative-semantic minus visuoperceptual conditions across subjects and significance map (green) from the correlation between change of naming and change of gray matter volume (Figure 4.2 *B*). Threshold: Uncorrected P<0.001. Same conventions as Figure 4.1

4.5 Discussion

Naming declined significantly in one third of the PPA patients over a one year period. Patients whose naming performance declined had significantly lower anterior temporal gray matter volumes at time of inclusion compared to patients who remained stable. Progression of anomia was associated with left posterior inferior temporal (BA 37) and right-sided temporal gray matter volume decrease (Fig. 4.2 *B*). The combination of cross-sectional (Fig. 4.2 *A*, *C*) and longitudinal (Fig. 4.2 *B*) findings suggests that atrophy associated with naming impairment progresses from anterior to posterior along the inferior temporal gyrus and from left to right.

From cross-sectional studies of PPA [44] [38], one might also expect frontal gray matter volume changes to be associated with language deterioration. However, in cross-sectional studies, frontal atrophy results mainly from group comparisons between patients with progressive non-fluent aphasia (PNFA) and normal controls [44] [38], whereas correlations between naming and gray matter volume predominantly implicate the temporal lobe, irrespective of clinical subtype PNFA or semantic dementia [44]. Clinical heterogeneity of PPA patients without comprehension deficit may also explain the absence of frontal changes [38] [238].

The degree of atrophy of the left anterior temporal lobe was predictive of a higher rate of naming decline (Fig. 4.1). This region corresponded to the main locus of atrophy associated with naming impairment cross-sectionally (Fig. 4.2 *A, C*). A similar disease mechanism is present in AD where medial temporal atrophy is predictive of memory decline [63] [275] [278] [276] [277] [187] [274]. This suggests that a higher degree of atrophy in brain regions of interest for a certain cognitive phenotype predicts a higher rate of cognitive deterioration during follow-up. The temporal relationship between the structural imaging findings and cognitive decline advocates the use of MRI as a prognostic tool on top of its use as a diagnostic tool.

The posterior temporal and contralateral extension of gray matter volume loss associated with naming decline during follow-up fits with the distribution of atrophy described in more advanced relative to milder stages of PPA in cross-sectional studies [41] [287] as well as in neuropathological studies [288]. In other neurodegenerative disorders such as MCI and AD, atrophic changes associated with cognitive decline have a more distributed pattern and include medial temporal cortex [274] [275], temporal neocortex and cingulate, parietal and orbitofrontal areas [273] [187] [283]. A relatively focal distribution of atrophy is one of the hallmarks of PPA [174] [288]. The finding that progression of atrophy is also spatially restricted, further explains why non-language domains remain largely unimpaired till more advanced disease stages [43]. The regional specificity of progression of atrophy in PPA is an important advantage in terms of its potential value as a biomarker for disease progression.

The correlation between naming decline and the rate of left posterior inferior temporal atrophy is in line with the critical role of left PITC in object naming. In other patient studies, lesions of left PITC as a result of occlusion of the left posterior cerebral artery [25] or electric stimulation of this area as part of a presurgical evaluation in patients with intractable epilepsy [289] both elicit object naming deficits [289]. Reperfusion of left PITC after stroke improves picture naming performance [290]. The absence of a correlation between gray matter volume changes of left PITC and change of the object decision task ($r = -0.02$) make object recognition problems unlikely as an explanation for the correlation with naming. This corroborates earlier functional imaging studies, in which left PITC is activated during object naming compared to object recognition tasks [291] [292] [145] and during name retrieval in response to auditory as well as to visual cues [293]. In addition to the correlation with naming decline, left PITC also correlated with change of performance on the single word comprehension task. This suggest that left PITC is involved in mapping the meaning of a concept to its name and vice versa. Our fMRI findings also confirm hypo-activity of left PITC in PPA during retrieval of the meaning of words or pictures [55]. Activity changes preceding gray matter volume changes may be explained by neuronal dysfunction preceding actual cell loss [294].

In conclusion, PPA patients with a higher degree of anterior temporal atrophy are at risk for an accelerated decline. This finding is clinically important in terms of counseling patients and caregivers. Progression of anomia is associated with gray matter volume loss of the left posterior inferior temporal cortex and right temporal cortex. The rate of atrophy provides us with a brain measure of disease progression and may be used for evaluating the effect of drugs intervention in PPA.

Chapter 5

Word reading and posterior temporal dysfunction in amnestic mild cognitive impairment

Cerebral cortex, In press, 2007
Mathieu Vandenbulcke[1,2], Ronald Peeters[3], Patrick Dupont[4], Paul Van Hecke[3], Rik Vandenberghe[1,5]
[1]Cognitive Neurology Laboratory, Experimental Neurology Division, Katholieke Universiteit Leuven, Belgium and [2]Psychiatry Department, [3]Radiology Department, [4]Nuclear Medicine Department, University Hospitals Gasthuisberg Leuven, Belgium.

5.1 Abstract

Patient studies that combine fMRI with chronometric analysis of language dysfunction may reveal the critical contribution of brain areas to language processes as well as shed light on disease pathogenesis. In amnestic mild cognitive impairment (MCI), a prodromal stage of Alzheimer's disease, we examined whether the brain system for associative-semantic judgements with words or with pictures is affected and how this relates to off-line chronometric analysis of word reading and picture naming. A consecutive memory-clinic based series of 13 amnestic MCI patients participated as well as 13 matched controls. One area, the lower bank of the posterior third of the left superior temporal sulcus (STS), showed a significant group-by-task interaction: In controls, it was activated during the associative-semantic condition with words compared to the visuoperceptual control condition but not when the same tasks were compared with pictures as input. In MCI, this word-specific activation was significantly reduced. Response amplitude correlated (r=0.90) with the steepness of the slope of the time-accuracy curve for word reading. Our data provide converging evidence for a critical contribution of the lower bank of the left posterior STS to mapping word form onto word meaning (lexical-semantic retrieval).

5.2 Introduction

In cognitive neuroscience, patient studies have an important place because they may provide insight into the pathogenesis of cognitive dysfunction but also because from the consequences of regional brain dysfunction essential information can be derived about the critical nature of the contribution of specific brain regions to cognitive processes [295]. In this study of the brain substrate of language and semantic memory, we combined fMRI in healthy controls with fMRI in patients. We examined how pathological alterations of fMRI activity patterns related to chronometric measures of word reading and picture naming [295].

We selected a patient population who did not show a clinical language or semantic memory deficit according to conventional neuropsychological testing at the moment of testing but were at risk for developing clinically evident language or semantic memory problems over the years to come. Recently, brain alterations that precede the dementia stage of Alzheimer's disease have evoked a lot of interest. In memory-clinic based cohorts, a valid clinical approximation of this pre-dementia stage is "amnestic mild cognitive impairment" (MCI) [56] [296]. Amnestic MCI is clinically defined by the presence of a subjective complaint of memory decline, corroborated by an informant, objective impairment of episodic memory on routine neuropsychological assessment and minimal impact upon instrumental activities of daily living (IADL) [296]. Other cognitive domains are relatively preserved or only mildly affected, in which case the designation "amnestic MCI-multi-domain" has been proposed [296]. In memory-clinic based cohorts, when criteria are strictly applied and alternative causes are rigorously excluded, approximately 80% of patients clinically diagnosed with amnestic MCI convert to probable AD within six years [296]. The clinical condition of amnestic MCI provides us with a time window to study AD-related changes of the language and semantic memory system that chronologically precede the dementia stage [56]. fMRI studies in amnestic MCI until now have principally focussed on episodic memory and on medial temporal volumes of interest [82] [83] [85] [86] [84].

We addressed two questions: First, is the network for language and semantic memory altered in amnestic MCI despite apparent preservation clinically and are word-specific regions mainly affected or components of the semantic memory system that are independent of input modality (words or pictures)? Two mechanisms for the word finding problems in probable AD have been proposed: Degradation of the semantic memory system [70] [76] [80] [297] or a word-specific semantic access deficit [298] [299] [300]. If the semantic memory system is degraded, one would expect that a deficit is present not only for words but also when pictures are used as input-modality. Indeed, AD patients who fail to name a picture are also deficient in retrieval of knowledge about the picture, even when tested by non-verbal means [70] [76]. On the basis of these findings in probable AD, we predicted that amnestic MCI would be associated with changes in input-modality independent semantic processing areas rather than word-specific processing areas.

As our second research question, we asked how regional dysfunction measured using fMRI relates to off-line chronometric analysis of word reading and picture naming. Our chronometric analysis was based on a time-accuracy approach that allowed to decompose word reading and picture naming into different processes [161] [162]. We varied word or picture exposure duration and determined accuracy as a function of stimulus duration. Three measures can be derived for each individual's time-accuracy curve: The time of onset of the rising phase, the steepness of the slope and the accuracy asymptote [161] [162]. These parameters reflect different processes. E.g. a delay of the onset of the word reading curve may arise from early visual identification problems that impair letter identification. At the other end, a lowering of the asymptote of the word reading curve may arise from speech output problems, such as phonological output, phonetic or articulatory deficits [247]. When onset or asymptote of the time-accuracy curves do not differ between groups but the slope does, time-sensitive processes are impaired that facilitate word reading and lie in between the early visual identification processes and speech output processes. In a reading experiment with regular words, these time-sensitive facilitatory processes include lexical assembly (phoneme-to-grapheme conversion) and lexical retrieval processes (orthographic-lexical, lexical-semantic and lexical-phonological retrieval) [301] [295] [147] [247]. We correlated the parameters that define the time-accuracy curve with fMRI response amplitude in those areas that were affected in the patients.

5.3 Subjects and Methods

5.3.1 Subjects

A consecutive series of 13 patients (8 men, 5 women) who were recruited via the memory clinic, University Hospital Gasthuisberg, Leuven, participated. They fulfilled the clinical diagnostic criteria for amnestic Mild Cognitive Impairment (MCI) [296]. Patients were between 55 and 76 years of age (mean 65.8, s.d. 6.8 years), mean educational level was 12.7 years (s.d. 2.7) and mean modified Edinburgh Inventory handedness score +88.7. Memory impairment was the primary reason for attending the memory clinic in all patients and memory decline was confirmed by an informant and by a routine clinical neuropsychological evaluation. Other cognitive domains and instrumental activities of daily living were relatively preserved so that a diagnosis of clinically probable AD [243] [302] could not be made. Clinical Dementia Rating (CDR) scale [256] was 0.5 in each of the patients, with a mean memory score of 0.58 (s.d. 0.18) We excluded patients who had significant vascular lesions on clinical Fluid-Attenuated Recovery (FLAIR) MRI sequences. All subjects were formally psychiatrically assessed to exclude mood or anxiety disorders as a cause of the memory complaint. All were free from cognitive enhancing or other psychotropic medication.

The MCI patients were compared with 13 cognitively intact controls, matched for gender (8 men, 5 women), age (mean age 65.9, s.d. 6.3, range 56-77 years), educational level (12.9 years, s.d. 2.6), handedness (modified Edinburgh Inventory +87.4) and vascular risk factors. The controls were selected from a cohort of elderly cognitively intact subjects recruited through advertisement in a regional newspaper. Controls did not have any memory complaints and had no history of significant neurological or psychiatric illness.

After complete description of the study to the subjects, written informed consent was obtained in accordance with the Declaration of Helsinki. The study protocol was approved by the Ethical Committee, University Hospital Gasthuisberg, Leuven.

After inclusion, MCI patients and controls underwent a standard neuropsychological research protocol (Table 5.1). Controls as well as all MCI patients except one (case 7) also underwent apoE genotyping after inclusion in the study. The MCI group comprised 5 apolipoprotein E ϵ4 heterozygotes (41%) and 1 homozygote (8%), the control group 3 apolipoprotein E ϵ4 heterozygotes (23%) and no homozygotes.

5.3.2 Neuropsychological protocol

Language was assessed by means of the validated Dutch versions of the Aachen Aphasie Test [101] and the Verbal Assocation test of the Psycholinguistic Assessment of Language Processing in Aphasia (PALPA) [103]. Episodic memory was tested by means of the Auditory Verbal Learning Test and the Rey Visual Design Learning Test. Other cognitive domains were tested by means of the Trail Making Test (TMT), the Raven's Coloured Progressive Matrices (CPM), the Number Location test of the Visual Object and Space Perception Battery [107] and the Object decision test of the Birmingham Object Recognition Battery [106]. The Functional Activities Questionnaire (FAQ) [303] and the CDR total score [256] were also included.

5.3.3 fMRI experiment: Stimuli and tasks

Stimuli were projected from a Barco 6300 LCD projector (1280x1024 pixels) onto a screen 28 cm in front of the subjects' eyes. The experiment was conducted using Superlab for PC version 2.0 (Cedrus, Phoenix, AR, USA).

The design of the fMRI experiment was factorial [5]. The first factor, task, had two levels: Associative-semantic versus visuoperceptual judgment. The second factor, input modality, also had two levels: Pictures versus printed words. The associative semantic condition was derived from the Pyramids and Palm Trees test (PPT) [128] (Fig. 5.1*A*).

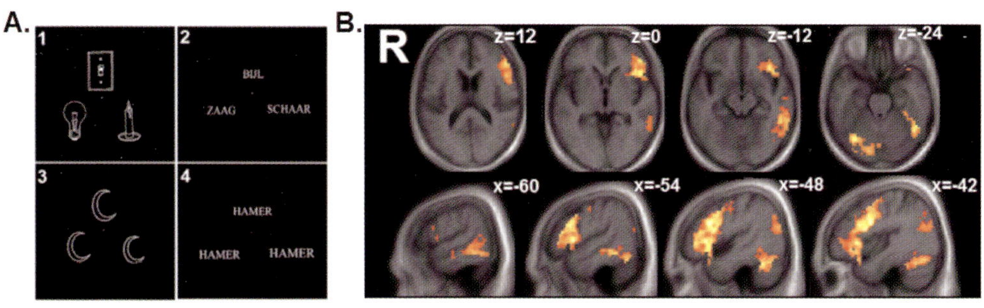

Figure 5.1: **A.** Stimuli and tasks. *1,2.* Associative-semantic task with pictures (*1*) and with words (*2*) (translation: Sample stimulus: Axe; Test stimuli: Saw and scissors). *3,4.* Visuoperceptual task with pictures (*3*) or words (*4*) (translation: Hammer). **B.** Search volume obtained from the subtraction associative-semantic minus visuoperceptual conditions across groups (contrast *1*). *Threshold:* Uncorrected $P<0.001$. X and z: Talairach coordinates (in mm).

During a trial, a triplet of stimuli was presented for 5250 ms, one stimulus on top (the sample stimulus) and one in each lower quadrant (the test stimuli), at 3.8 deg eccentricity, followed by a 1500 ms interval. Subjects had to press a left- or right-hand key depending on which of the two test stimuli matched the sample stimulus more closely in meaning. A given triplet was presented in either the picture (Fig. 5.1*A.1*) or the word format (Fig. 5.1*A.2*) and this was counterbalanced across subjects. In the visuoperceptual control condition, a picture (Fig. 5.1*A.3*) or word stimulus (Fig. 5.1*A.4*) was presented in three different sizes. Subjects had to press a left or right-hand key depending on which of the two test stimuli matched the sample stimulus more closely in size on the screen.

5.3.4 Image acquisition

A 1.5 tesla Siemens Sonata system (Siemens Medical Solutions, Erlangen, Germany) equipped with an 8-channel receive-only head coil (MRI Devices Corp., Waukesha, USA) provided a high-resolution MPRAGE T1-weighted structural volume as well as T2* echo-planar images (EPI) (42 sagittal slices; voxel size 3x3x3 mm^3; TE/TR 40/3000 ms). Usage of the GeneRalized Autocalibrating Partially Parallel Acquisitions (GRAPPA) method together with sagittal acquisition maximized sensitivity for anterior temporal activity changes and minimized susceptibility artifacts [177]. A total of 108 volumes were acquired during each run. Each run consisted of 3 replications of each of the 4 conditions. Each epoch, i.e. a block of trials of the same type, consisted of 4 trials (total duration 27 s). Subjects underwent 4 to 6 runs each.

5.3.5 Image analysis

We used Statistical Parametric Mapping 2002. Head motion parameters did not differ between groups ($P \succ 0.9$). After realignment, reslicing and normalisation [180] the EPI volumes were spatially smoothed using a 6 mm FWHM isotropic Gaussian kernel. A high-pass filter of 216 s was applied and a low-pass filter consisting of a canonical hemodynamic response function (HRF). The epoch-related response was modeled by a canonical HRF, convolved with a boxcar.

A t statistic for the parameter estimates was generated for each subject for the following contrasts

1. (Associative-semantic task with words + Associative-semantic task with pictures) - (Visuoperceptual task with words + Visuoperceptual task with pictures)

2. Associative-semantic task with words - Visuoperceptual task with words

3. Associative-semantic task with pictures - Visuoperceptual task with pictures

4. (Associative-semantic task with words + Visuoperceptual task with words) - (Associative-semantic task with pictures + visuoperceptual task with pictures), and inversely

5. (Associative-semantic task with words - Visuoperceptual task with words) - (Associative-semantic task with pictures - visuoperceptual task with pictures), and inversely

The t map was subsequently transformed to a Z map. The data did not show any outlier or clustering [183]. We weighted the individuals' contrast images for the total number of runs per subject and entered the significance maps into a second level analysis. Using a one-sample t test, we first defined our search volume: We determined where the associative semantic condition yielded higher activity than the visuoperceptual condition (contrast *1*) across subjects at an uncorrected $P \prec 0.001$. Within this search volume, we determined where the images for each of the above contrasts (contrasts *1-5*) differed between controls and MCI patients. We used a two-sample t test with a voxel-level significance threshold set at $P \prec 0.05$ corrected for the search volume.

We wanted to exclude that between-group differences in gray matter volume contributed to functional activity differences. We conducted an optimized voxel-based morphometric (VBM) analysis [184]. Using a two-sample t test we examined where gray matter volume differed between controls and MCI patients.

5.3.6 Chronometric experiment

In order to assess word or picture processing with higher sensitivity, we conducted a chronometric study. A trial consisted of a forward mask (200 ms duration), followed by a test stimulus (a word or a picture) which was immediately followed by a backward mask (200 ms duration). Word size was 1.5 deg and picture size 5.7 deg. Only regular words were used. Test stimulus presentation duration varied between 30, 45, 60, 90, 150, 200, 500 or 800 ms. Subjects were instructed to read the word or name the picture. Subjects received 320 trials in total. Each concept was presented once as a word and once as a picture in a counterbalanced order. For each individual, onset, slope and asymptote of the time-accuracy function for words and pictures were calculated by means of the following equation [161] [162]:

$$p = \begin{cases} c(1 - e^{(a-\Delta t)/b}) & \text{if } \Delta t \geq a \\ 0 & \text{if } 0 \leq \Delta t < a. \end{cases} \tag{5.1}$$

In this equation, p stands for the percentage of correctly answered items, which is a function of presentation time Δt. The curve described by Equation 1 is negatively accelerating, that is, it remains at zero up to a certain point in time (parameter a), where it starts to rise steeply, and it becomes less and less steep with advancing presentation time, flattening toward a horizontal asymptote (parameter c) [162]. The a parameter (the onset) represents the point on the time axis where performance starts to rise above zero. The c parameter (the asymptote) represents the level of performance a participant would reach if an unlimited amount of time were available. The b parameter (the rate of approach) represents the rate at which performance goes to the asymptote. Higher values of b indicate that the time-accuracy function is less steep, that is, participants with higher b values are slower in reaching the asymptotic level of performance than participants with lower b values. The b parameter presumably reflects the speed of deployment of the elaboration process, that is, the rate at which associations can be generated to the stimulus [162]. Goodness of fit was estimated as the sum of squared differences between the measured and calculated values (SSE).

Ten of the MCI patients (cases 1-3,5,6,8-10,12,13) and 10 matched controls participated in the chronometric study. After neuropsychological assessment and the fMRI session, our research protocol proved to be too demanding for cases 4, 7 and 11. These patients did not want to participate in the chronometric experiment, the last part of the initial evaluation.

We used Analysis of Variance (ANOVA) to compare word and picture identification parameters a, b and c between MCI patients and controls. We carried out a multiple linear regression analysis with fMRI response amplitude as outcome variable and the psychophysical word and picture identification parameters a, b and c as regressors. This analysis was restricted to a spherical volume of interest (radius 3 voxels) surrounding the voxels of peak differential activation between MCI and controls. The analysis was carried out on the data of the MCI patients only and was therefore independent of the voxel selection criterion. The significance map was thresholded at a voxel-level inference of $P \prec 0.05$ corrected for the spherical volume of interest.

5.3.7 Follow-up

During the first year of follow-up, case 7 (Table 5.1) died from an unrelated cause and case 11 (Table 5.1) withdrew consent. After 1 year, the 11 remaining patients and 11 matched controls underwent a clinical and neuropsychological re-evaluation and a repeat structural and functional MRI. Subjects were also re-evaluated clinically and neuropsychologically after the second year.

For the follow-up scans, we determined where the difference between the associative-semantic and the visuoperceptual conditions (contrast *1*) differed between patients and controls at the second time point (two-sample t test, significance threshold $P \prec 0.05$ corrected for the search volume).

5.4 Results

5.4.1 Neuropsychological data

As a group, patients performed significantly worse than controls on all measures of episodic memory performance (Student's t test for independent samples: $P \prec 0.05$; Table 5.1) but not in other cognitive domains. In each of the MCI individuals the score of at least one episodic memory task fell two standard deviations below the mean of our age- and education-matched controls (Table 5.1). In 8 subjects, performance in cognitive domains other than episodic memory was strictly preserved neuropsychologically. The remaining 5 subjects scored more than 2 standard deviations lower than our controls on one (case 9-11) or more non-episodic memory measures (case 12,13). These patients could be classified as amnestic MCI-multi-domain [296]. One patient (case 13) scored within the range of published age- and education-based norms on the Akense Afasie test [101] but just below two s.d. compared to our own matched controls.

5.4.2 Performance of the fMRI experiment

We conducted a three-factor repeated-measures Analysis of Variance of reaction times, accuracies and omissions, with stimulus modality and task as within-subject factors (two levels: pictures *versus* words and semantic *versus* visuoperceptual, respectively) and with group as between-subject factor (two levels: MCI *versus* controls) (Table 5.2 and Table 5.3).

Case	1	2	3	4	5	6	7	8	9	10	11	12	13	MCI mean (s.d.)	Controls mean (s.d.)	t
Age (years)	55	55	60	62	68	68	70	76	63	64	67	73	75	65.8 (6.8)	65.9 (6.3)	0.0
Education (years)	17	14	9	12	14	16	17	12	11	12	9	10	12	12.7 (2.7)	12.9 (2.6)	0.0
FAQ (/7)	**2**	**2**	**2**	**2**	**3**	**2**	**2**	**2**	**3**	**2**	**2**	**2**	**3**	**2.2** (0.4)	1.0 (0.0)	-9.8
Clinical Dementia Rating																
Global CDR (/3)	**0.5**	**0.5**	**0.5**	**0.5**	**0.5**	**0.5**	**0.5**	**0.5**	**0.5**	**0.5**	**0.5**	**0.5**	**0.5**	**0.5** (0)	0 (0)	-14.0
Sum of the boxes(/18)	**2.5**	**0.5**	**1**	**0.5**	**2.5**	**1**	**1.5**	**0.5**	**3**	**2**	**1.5**	**1.5**	**1**	**1.5** (0.85)	0 (0)	-5.2
Auditory Verbal Learning Test																
Learning (/75)	**33**	48	**35**	43	**31**	**34**	49	**36**	**31**	**23**	**29**	**27**	**17**	**33.7** (9.2)	50.1 (6.5)	5.4
Recall (/15)	**5**	8	**4**	**6**	**0**	**5**	9	**2**	**5**	**1**	**6**	**1**	**0**	**4.2** (3.3)	11.2 (1.7)	6.6
% Recall	**71**	**61**	**50**	**50**	**0**	**55**	**75**	**28**	**71**	**20**	**75**	**20**	**0**	**47.3** (31.4)	90.1 (7.4)	4.7
Recognition (/15)	**8**	14	**12**	**13**	14	**12**	14	**13**	14	**4**	15	**7**	**6**	**11.3** (3.7)	14.6 (0.6)	3.0
Rey Visual Design Learning Test																
Recognition (/15)	**9**	14	**11**	13	**5**	14	13	13	12	**9**	14	**8**	13	**11.4** (2.9)	14.0 (1.4)	3.1
Aachen Aphasie Test																
Naming (/120)	119	116	117	115	117	119	120	109	114	110	116	115	**105**	114.7 (4.3)	117.2 (4.4)	1.6
Comprehension (/120)	116	119	105	117	112	117	111	112	111	109	112	115	109	112.7 (3.9)	113.6 (5.4)	1.4
Auditory word-picture matching (/30)	29	30	24	30	27	30	28	**25**	26	30	23	30	26	27.5 (2.5)	28.7 (1.8)	1.4
Auditory sentence-picture matching (/30)	30	30	28	30	27	30	27	30	27	26	29	27	30	27.8 (2.8)	28.7 (1.8)	1.1
Visual word-picture matching (/30)	30	29	**26**	29	29	30	30	27	28	28	30	29	27	28.6 (1.3)	28.8 (1.0)	0.5
Visual sentence-picture matching (/30)	27	30	27	28	29	27	26	30	30	25	30	29	26	28.0 (1.8)	27.8 (2.1)	-0.3
Spontaneous speech (/30)	30	30	30	30	30	30	30	29	30	30	29	30	29	29.7 (0.4)	29.8 (0.4)	0.5
Communicative behavior (/5)	5	5	5	5	5	5	5	5	5	5	5	5	5	5.0 (0.0)	5.0 (0.0)	0.0
Articulation (/5)	5	5	5	5	5	5	5	5	5	5	5	5	5	5.0 (0.0)	5.0 (0.0)	0.0
Automatized language (/5)	5	5	5	5	5	5	5	5	5	5	5	5	5	5.0 (0.0)	5.0 (0.0)	0.0
Semantic structure (/5)	5	5	5	5	5	5	5	**4**	5	5	5	5	**4**	4.8 (0.4)	4.9 (0.3)	0.6
Phonological structure (/5)	5	5	5	5	5	5	5	5	5	5	5	5	5	5.0 (0.0)	5.0 (0.0)	0.0
Syntactic structure (/5)	5	5	5	5	5	5	5	5	5	5	**4**	5	5	4.9 (0.3)	4.9 (0.3)	0.0
Reading (/30)	30	30	30	30	30	30	30	30	30	30	30	30	30	30 (0.0)	30 (0.0)	0.0
Writing (/30)	30	30	30	29	30	30	28	30	30	30	28	28	30	29.4 (0.8)	29.5 (0.8)	0.8
Repetition (/150)	150	150	146	150	148	147	150	150	150	149	146	149	**139**	148.0 (3.1)	148.9 (1.7)	0.4
PALPA (/30)	30	29	29	29	29	27	30	29	30	28	27	29	25	28.5 (1.4)	28.4 (1.7)	-0.2
TMT	2.0	2.6	3.2	1.8	3.2	2.7	1.7	2.3	2.7	2.6	3.0	**4.2**	3.2	2.71 (0.68)	2.55 (0.63)	-2.2
CPM (/36)	36	36	27	36	29	34	35	33	30	30	**23**	**19**	29	30.5 (5.3)	32.4 (2.7)	1.8
Number location (/10)	8	10	10	9	10	10	7	9	9	8	9	10	10	9.1 (0.9)	9.4 (0.7)	1.2
Object decision (/64)	58	57	57	57	55	56	57	55	**47**	**51**	57	55	**47**	54.5 (3.8)	57.8 (2.0)	2.3

Table 5.1: Neuropsychological individual and group data. Individual data: *Bold*: 2 standard deviations lower than average of our age- and education-matched controls. Group data: *Bold*: $P \prec 0.05$ corrected for multiple comparisons.

Subjects performed the visuoperceptual task faster than the semantic task ($F(1,24)=132$, $P \prec 0.00001$), more accurately ($F(1,24)=61.5$, $P \prec 0.00001$) and with fewer omissions ($F(1,24)=7.8$, $P \prec 0.01$). Subjects responded faster during the word compared to the picture conditions ($F(1,24)=22.7$, $P \prec 0.0001$) and more accurately ($F(1,24)=11.7$, $P \prec 0.01$). The number of omissions did not differ significantly between word and picture conditions ($F(1,24)=2.9$, $P=0.1$).

Reaction times ($F(1,24)=0.8$, $P=0.3$), accuracies ($F(1,24)=2.5$, $P=0.1$) or omissions ($F(1,24)=1.8$, $P=0.2$) did not differ significantly between groups, although the MCI patients tended to be slower and less accurate and omit more responses than the control group (Table 5.2). There were no significant interactions between group and task, between group and modality. There were no three way interaction between modality, task and group for accuracies ($F(1,24)=0.006$, $P=0.93$), reaction times ($F(1,24)=0.014$, $P=0.90$) or omissions ($F(1,24)=0.34$, $P=0.56$).

5.4.3 fMRI data

Across groups, the contrast between the associative-semantic conditions and the visuoperceptual conditions (contrast *1*) activated a distributed left-hemispheric system (Fig. 5.1*B*) replicating previous results [5]. This activity map was used as our search volume to detect between-group differences for contrasts *1-5*.

The activity map obtained by the contrast of the associative semantic conditions minus the visuoperceptual conditions (contrast *1*) differed between controls and patients in one region:

	Reaction time (ms)		Accuracy (% correct)		Omissions (%)	
	MCI	Controls	MCI	Controls	MCI	Controls
Semantic(P)	3028 (493)	2962 (464)	80.1 (7.5)	81.4 (8.3)	5.9 (6.1)	6.4 (5.7)
Semantic(W)	2947 (694)	2819 (406)	84.6 (9.3)	87.6 (6.8)	7.3 (9.3)	2.4 (6.8)
Visuoperceptual(P)	2692 (673)	2475 (529)	87.4 (9.0)	91.0 (6.5)	6.0 (8.2)	2.4 (6.1)
Visuoperceptual(W)	2381 (406)	2136 (446)	88.0 (10.0)	92.4 (7.2)	5.1 (6.1)	1.3 (4.6)

Table 5.2: Performance parameters obtained in the fMRI experiment (mean (s.d.)). *Abbreviations:* Semantic(P): Associative-semantic task with pictures; Semantic(W): Associative-semantic task with words; Visuoperceptual(P): Visuoperceptual task with pictures: Visuoperceptual(W): Visuoperceptual task with words.

Case	1	2	3	4	5	6	7	8	9	10	11	12	13	Controls mean (s.d.)
Accuracy (% correct)														
Semantic(P)	84	89	80	90	74	92	85	76	81	80	73	70	67	81.4 (8.3)
Semantic(W)	90	89	85	95	85	90	100	90	78	85	**68**	75	**71**	87.6 (6.8)
Visuoperceptual(P)	87	98	90	93	**76**	93	98	94	87	87	78	88	**67**	91.0 (6.5)
Visuoperceptual(W)	94	96	85	96	83	98	98	97	89	89	78	*71*	**70**	92.4 (7.2)
Reaction time (ms)														
Semantic(P)	2785	3269	2711	2409	3577	2658	3151	2635	3176	2820	2488	3713	**3980**	2962 (464)
Semantic(W)	2807	3041	2956	2545	3018	2710	2883	2298	2589	2950	2689	3554	**4279**	2819 (406)
Visuoperceptual(P)	2387	2446	2322	2157	3304	1944	3201	1899	2774	2807	2071	**3876**	**3810**	2475 (529)
Visuoperceptual(W)	2157	2272	2318	1941	2671	1894	2676	1971	2319	2438	2122	2880	**3294**	2136 (446)

Table 5.3: Individual performance parameters during the fMRI experiment. *Bold*: 2 standard deviations lower than average of our age- and education-matched controls. Same conventions as in Table 5.2

The posterior third of the lower bank of the left superior temporal sulcus (Fig. 5.2*A*, 5.3*A*). The group-by-task interaction was significant (-60,-42,0, ext. 21, Z=4.32, P≺0.05 corrected for the search volume). When we restricted the analysis to the word conditions only (contrast *2*), the group-by-task interaction remained significant (-63, -39, 0, ext. 18, Z=4.10, P≺0.05 corrected for the search volume) (Fig. 5.3*C* versus *D red* versus *magenta*) but not when the analysis was restricted to the picture conditions only (contrast *3*; uncorr. P≻ 0.01) (Fig. 5.3*C* versus *D blue* versus *cyan*).

In controls, this region was activated during the associative-semantic condition with words in comparison to the visuoperceptual condition with words (-60, -42, 0, Z=4.58, uncorr. P≺0.00001; Fig. 5.3*C red* versus *magenta*) but not when the same tasks were compared with pictures as input (uncorr. P≻0.01; Fig. 5.3*C blue* versus *cyan*). The posterior STS voxels that showed a modality-by-task interaction at uncorr. P≺0.001 are shown in Fig. 5.3*B* in blue. These word-specific voxels partially overlapped with the voxels that showed a group-by-task interaction (Fig. 5.3*B blue* versus *red*).

Inferior to the voxels that showed word-specific activation (Fig. 5.3*B blue*) a cluster of voxels showed input modality-independent activation during the associative-semantic minus the visuoperceptual conditions regardless of input-modality, words or pictures (Fig. 5.3*B green*) (conjunction analysis [304] -63,-39,-6, Z=4.87, P≺0.05 corrected for the entire brain). This replicates our previous findings in the left posterior middle temporal gyrus [5]. These input modality-independent voxels are shown in Fig. 5.3*B* in green.

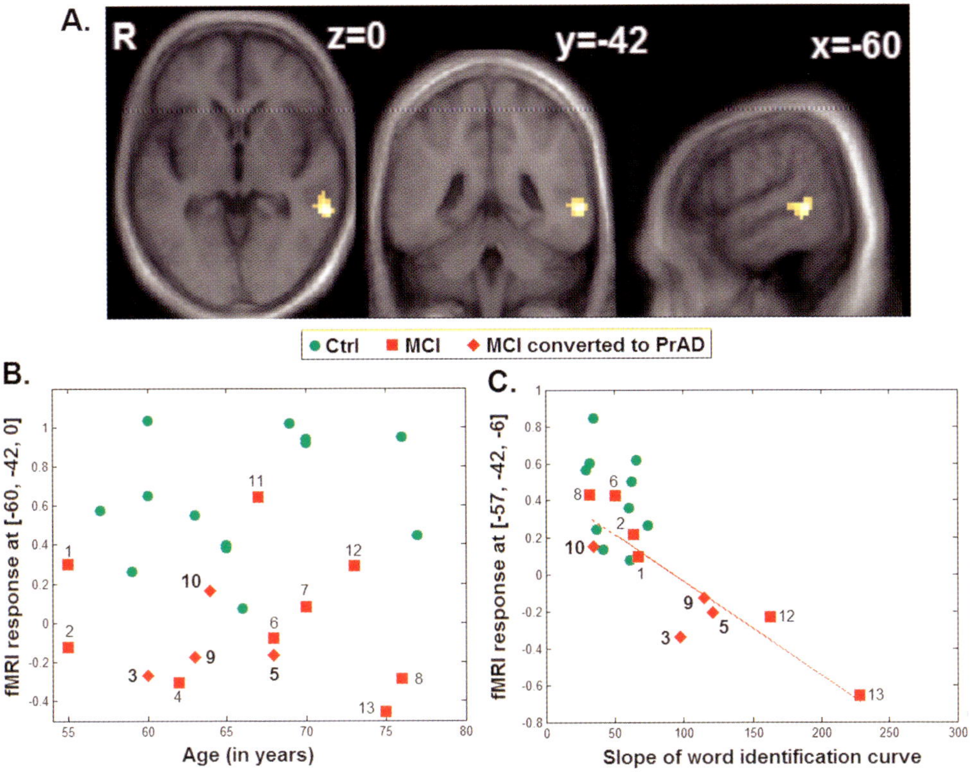

Figure 5.2: **A.** Map of higher activity in controls compared to MCI during the associative semantic conditions compared to the visuoperceptual conditions (group-by-task interaction). Superposition onto the group-averaged structural brain MRI. Uncorrected $P<0.001$. **B.** Individual fMRI responses in the peak of the cluster depicted in Fig. 5.2*A*. X axis: Age; Y axis: Percentage signal change in the peak voxel of the cluster depicted in Fig. 5.2*A*. Each datapoint corresponds to one individual. *Green*: Controls; *Red*: MCI; *Diamonds:* Converters. Indices correspond to those used in Table 5.1. **C.** Correlation between the slope (psychophysical parameter *b*) of the word identification curve (Fig. 5.4*A*) and the fMRI response amplitude (% BOLD signal change) in posterior STS (Fig. 5.2*A*). Same conventions as in *A*.

Apart from the posterior superior temporal sulcus, no other brain areas showed a between-group difference of activity for any of the contrasts tested (contrasts 1-5) (uncorrected $P>0.005$). We did not find any regions where activity was higher in MCI compared to controls in the current study. VBM did not reveal any differences in gray matter volume between patients and normals in posterior temporal cortex (uncorrected $P>0.05$). There was no correlation between performance of the fMRI task and BOLD activity in the posterior temporal cortex (uncorr. $P>0.01$).

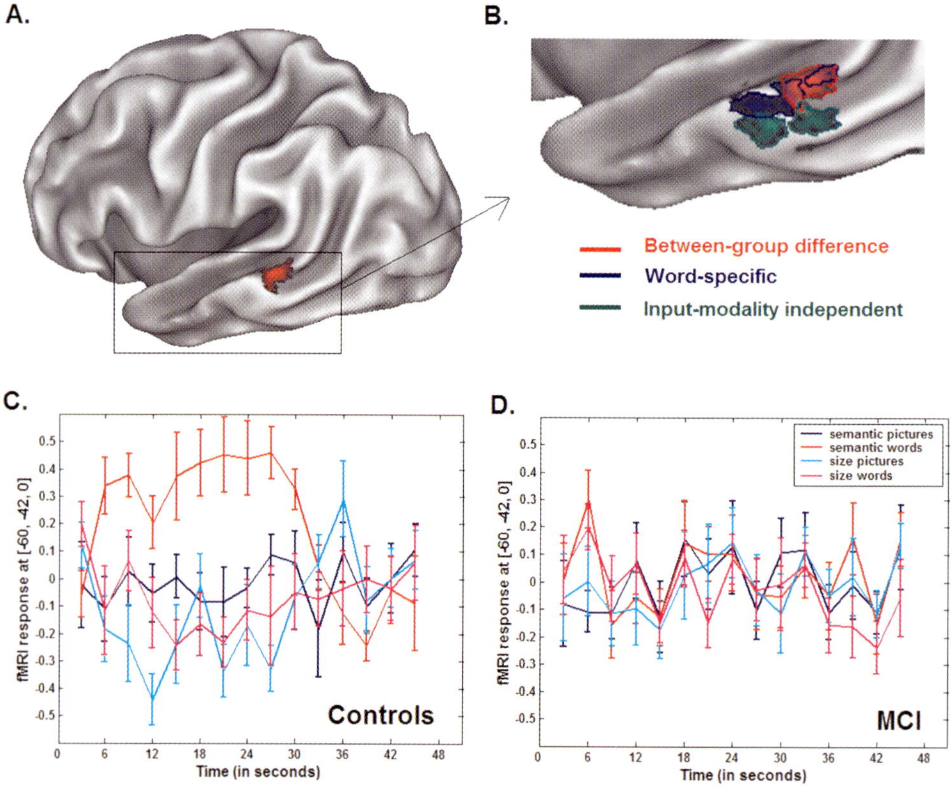

Figure 5.3: **A.** Map of higher activity in controls compared to MCI during the associative semantic conditions compared to the visuoperceptual conditions (group-by-task interaction). Uncorrected $P<0.001$. Superposition onto a standard brain using CARET software (lateral view) (Washington University School of Medicine, Department of Anatomy and Neurobiology, http://brainmap.wustl.edu). **B.** Superposition of three activity maps. *Red*: Group-by-task interaction: Higher activity in controls than in MCI during the associative-semantic compared to the visuoperceptual tasks. *Blue:* Control subjects: Task-by-modality interaction (contrast *5*): Higher activity during the associative-semantic compared to the visuoperceptual task with words than with pictures. *Green:* Control subjects: Conjunction analysis: Higher activity during the associative-semantic compared to the visuoperceptual task with words (contrast *2*) as well as with pictures (contrast *3*). Uncorrected $P<0.001$. **C.** Activity time course averaged over the control subjects in the peak voxel of the cluster depicted in Fig. 5.3*A* during the 4 types of epoch (epoch duration 27 s). *Red:* Associative-semantic judgment with words. *Blue:* Associative-semantic judgment with pictures. *Magenta:* Visuoperceptual judgment with words. *Cyan:* Visuoperceptual judgment with pictures. X axis: Time in s; Y axis: % BOLD signal change. **D.** Activity time course averaged over the MCI subjects in the peak voxel of the cluster depicted in Fig. 5.3*A*. Same conventions as in *C*.

5.4.4 Chronometric data *versus* fMRI

	Words				Pictures			
	MCI		Controls		MCI		Controls	
	mean	s.d.	mean	s.d.	mean	s.d.	mean	s.d.
Onset	55.8	32.2	39.7	14.8	75.6	30.3	59.7	19.9
Slope	**97.5**	61.9	**50.8**	15.4	125.5	76.5	92.1	27.5
Asymptote	91.8	10.7	98.6	1.9	77.7	12.9	85.3	12.3

Table 5.4: Psychophysical experiment. Parameters a (onset), b (steepness of slope) and c (asymptote) of the time-accuracy curves (mean (s.d.)). Lower values of b mean that the slope is steeper. *Bold*: Significant between-group difference at $P \prec 0.05$.

The slope (parameter b) of the time-accuracy function for words was significantly steeper in controls than in MCI ($F(1,18)=5.3$, $P \prec 0.05$) (Fig. 5.4*A*; Table 5.4). The slope for picture identification did not differ significantly between groups ($F(1,18)=1.6$, $P=0.2$) (Fig. 5.4*B*; Table 5.4). Onset (parameter a) ($F(1,18)=0.7$, $P=0.4$) or plateau (parameter c) ($F(1,18)=3.8$, $P=0.07$) of the word reading curve and onset or plateau for picture identification ($F(1,18)=2.8$, $P=0.1$ and $F(1,18)=0.6$, $P=0.4$, respectively) did not differ significantly between groups.

In order to evaluate whether case 13 (Fig. 5.4*A*) disproportionately influenced the group differences, we removed it from analysis: The difference of the steepness of the slope of the time-accuracy curve for word reading between MCI and controls remained significant ($F(1,17)=4.6$, $P \prec 0.05$).

Within a volume of interest centered around the activity peak in the posterior STS a significant and strong correlation existed between fMRI response amplitude and the steepness of the slope of the time-accuracy curve for word reading (-57,-42,-6, $Z=3.57$, r=-0.90, corrected $P \prec 0.05$) (Fig. 5.2*C*). No correlation was found within this volume with the other parameters of this curve or with psychophysical parameters of the time-accuracy curve for picture identification (-57,-39,-3, $Z=1.31$, r=-0.44, uncorr. $P \succ 0.05$).

5.4.5 Follow-up data

Within the first year 3 patients (case 5,9,10) converted from CDR 0.5 to CDR 1 and fulfilled criteria for probable AD after the first year. One additional patient (case 3) converted within the second year. Three of the converters (cases 3,5,9) had a word identification slope at initial evaluation that was less steep than any of the controls (Fig. 5.4*A*) as well as posterior STS activity below that seen in controls at initial scanning (Fig. 5.2*B,C*).

The fMRI data collected after the first year confirmed that the left posterior superior temporal sulcus was significantly less active during the associative-semantic compared to the visuoperceptual condition in the patients (converters and non-converters) compared to the controls (Fig. 5.5 *yellow*). Again, the task-by-group interaction was significant in the lower bank of the left posterior superior temporal sulcus (-63,-42,3, ext. 55, $Z=4.03$, corr. $P=0.05$)

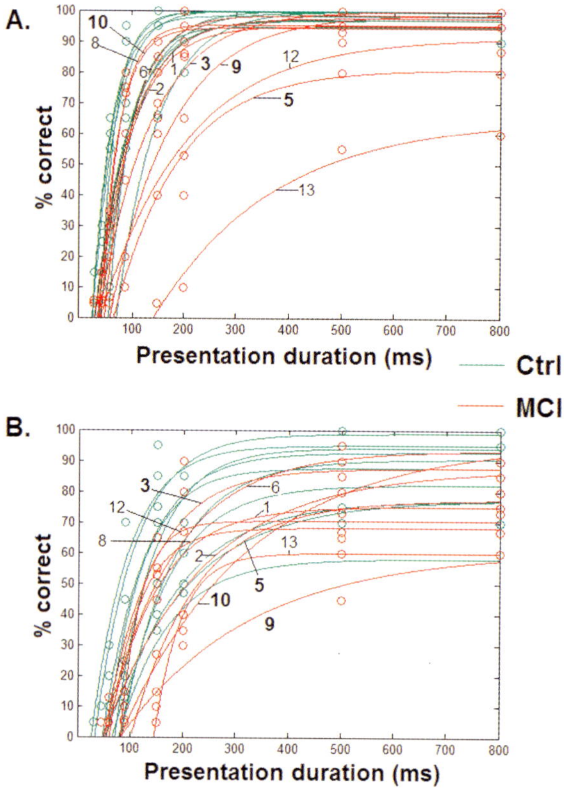

Figure 5.4: Chronometric experiment. **A.** Time-accuracy curve for word reading. X axis: Word presentation duration. Y axis: % correct responses. Each circle corresponds to an individual's mean accuracy at a given stimulus duration. *Red*: MCI. The indices identify the MCI individual and correspond to those used in Table 5.1. *Green*: Controls. *Bold:* Converter. **B.** Time-accuracy curve for picture naming. X axis: Picture presentation duration. Same conventions as in *A*.

(Fig. 5.5 *yellow*). A conjunction analysis (Nichols *et al.*, 2005) confirmed that the between-group differences overlapped between the two time points (-60,-39,0, ext. 30, Z=3.91, uncorr. $P<0.0001$) (Fig. 5.5 *yellow* versus *red*).

5.5 Discussion

Using fMRI we dissected left posterior temporal cortex and discerned two functionally distinct but juxtaposed regions (Fig. 5.3*B*): The lower bank of the posterior superior temporal sulcus, which is activated during associative semantic judgements with words specifically (Fig. 5.3*B*

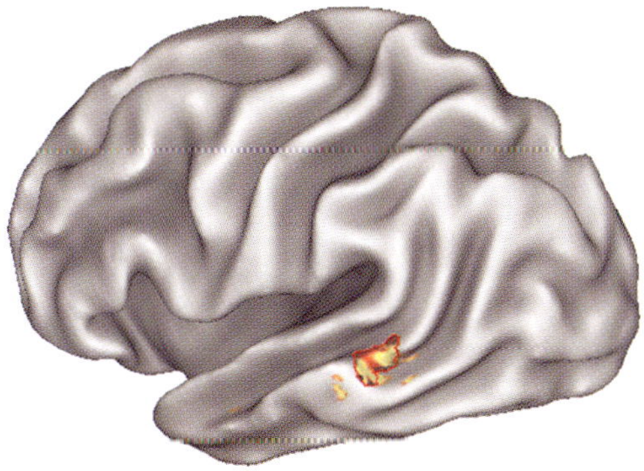

Figure 5.5: Map of higher activity in controls compared to MCI during the associative semantic compared to visuoperceptual conditions after 1 year follow-up (*yellow*) (group-by-task interaction). This map is superimposed onto the map obtained at the initial assessment (*red*). Uncorrected $P \prec 0.001$.

blue), and the middle temporal gyrus, which is activated during associative-semantic judgements regardless of input-modality, words or pictures (Fig. 5.3*B green*). Using a time-accuracy approach, we decomposed the reading process in a group of patients with amnestic MCI and demonstrated a change in the slope of the time-accuracy curve for written word identification. Amnestic MCI was also associated with dysfunction of the left posterior superior temporal sulcus, the word-specific processing region (Fig. 5.3*B red*). Hypo-activity of left posterior STS correlated inversely with the steepness of the slope of the time-accuracy curve for word reading (Fig. 5.2*C*).

The associative-semantic condition with words differed between groups not only in comparison to the visuoperceptual conditions but also in comparison to the associative-semantic condition with pictures (Fig. 5.3*C,D*). The most parsimonious explanation is a change during the associative-semantic condition with words rather than activity increases in the three other conditions of our factorial design. We did not include a low-level resting state condition as a reference because even the simplest baseline condition is associated with organized functional brain activity [134] which may itself be affected by disease [135].

Epidemiological studies based on primary care settings have suggested that mild cognitive impairment is a heterogeneous and unstable construct with poor predictive value [305]. Key differences between the Larrieu *et al.* (2002) [305] study and ours is the rigorous and prospective application of the Petersen *et al.* (2004) [296] criteria of amnestic MCI, strict exclusion criteria as well as patient recruitment via a memory clinic. Under these conditions, amnestic MCI constitutes a reasonable clinical approximation of incipient AD [56] [296]. The homogeneity of our subject sample is testified by the between-subject consistency of our random-effects fMRI results (Fig. 5.2*B*). Following inclusion we characterized our MCI sample genetically. Our MCI group contained more apolipoprotein E $\epsilon 4$ allele heterozygotes and homozygotes than the control group did, as one would expect in an AD risk group. During the first 2 years, 30.8% of the MCI group (cases 3,5,9,10) converted to probable AD, but none of the controls, confirming that AD risk was substantially higher in our amnestic MCI patients than in controls [296]. Five out of 13 MCI patients showed subtle changes in cognitive domains other than episodic memory. This subtype of amnestic MCI has sometimes been designated amnestic MCI-multi-domain [296]. This condition may carry a higher risk of conversion to AD than purely amnestic MCI [306].

In a previous reaction time study of written word identification in MCI [307], slowing of word identification speed predicted conversion to probable AD [307]. Our data provide an anatomical substrate for the word identification deficit in MCI [307]: The lower bank of the left posterior superior temporal sulcus (Fig. 5.2*A,C*). This localisation is compatible with the distribution of pathological depositions in Alzheimer's disease: The superior temporal sulcus is among the areas that show the highest density of neuritic plaques and neurofibrillary tangles in mild AD compared to normal controls [308].

In healthy controls the left posterior superior temporal sulcus (STS) is active during word reading in comparison to picture naming [309] [145] or in comparison to rest [310] and also when subjects attend to semantic relationships between semantically related written words compared to phonological relationships between rhyming words [311]. According to a seminal paper on word comprehension and retrieval [150], the left posterior and middle superior temporal sulcus showed higher activity when subjects compared the meaning of auditorily presented words but also when they generated verbs that were semantically appropriate to a presented concrete noun [150]. Its role in word comprehension as well as word generation was subsequently confirmed in several follow-up experiments [55] [11]. Our patient study complements these studies by demonstrating the critical nature of the contribution of the left posterior superior temporal sulcus to word reading (Fig. 5.2*C*). Processes specifically related to visual modality of word presentation, such as grapheme-to-phoneme conversion [301] or orthographic-lexical activation [147], are unlikely as an explanation since the posterior STS also responds to auditorily presented words [152] [312] [313]. Two possible explanations for STS activation as well as the change of steepness of slope remain: Lexical-semantic or lexical-phonological processing [295] [147] [247]. In our opinion, a lexical-semantic deficit is the more likely cause: Posterior STS is active when subjects carry out an associative-semantic task with words but not with pictures (Fig. 5.3*C,D*). This fits with a role in mapping word form onto word meaning (lexical-semantic retrieval [314]. Lexical-semantic retrieval also facilitates word identification [295]. This interpretation is in line with previous patient lesion studies that implicate the posterior temporal cortex in the two-way mapping between word form and word meaning [315] [316] [317] [318] [319] as well as functional imaging in healthy controls [311]. An alternative account of the left posterior STS findings lies at the level of lexical-phonological processing [320] [152] [321]. Strictly speaking, this possibility cannot be excluded since phonological and lexical-semantic processing may closely interact with each other and both may have a facilitatory effect on word identification as well as on associative-semantic tasks with words.

In probable AD single word reading problems have been principally attributed to a lexical-semantic retrieval deficit [322] [299] [323] [300] or a degradation of semantic representations [75] [76] [78] [32] [80] [81] [297]. We presented converging evidence for a word-specific role of STS. Our findings therefore strongly support an account in terms of a lexical retrieval problem rather than semantic degradation. On the basis of the current study in MCI and previous studies of semantic memory in probable AD [87] [88] we propose that, as the disease progresses to the stage of clinically probable AD, damage extends from word-specific processing regions, such as the posterior superior temporal sulcus, into modality-independent semantic processing areas such as the posterior middle temporal gyrus (Fig. 5.3*B*).

To conclude, left posterior temporal cortex contains two juxtaposed but functionally distinct regions, one in the lower bank of the superior temporal sulcus that is word-specific, one in the posterior middle temporal gyrus that is involved in semantic processing regardless of input-modality (Fig. 5.3*B* *blue* and *green*). Amnestic MCI is associated with dysfunction of the former area (Fig. 5.3*B* *blue* and *red*) leading to sub-clinical impairment of written word identification (Fig. 5.2*C*).

Chapter 6

Knowledge of visual attributes in the right hemisphere

Nature Neuroscience, 9, 964-970, 2006
Mathieu Vandenbulcke[1,2], Ronald Peeters[3], Katrien Fannes[4], Rik Vandenberghe[1,4]
[1]Cognitive Neurology Laboratory, K.U. Leuven, and Departments of [2]Psychiatry, [3]Radiology and [4]Neurology.

6.1 Abstract

Neurobiological theories of knowledge processing are biased towards the language dominant hemisphere. Does the right hemisphere critically contribute to knowledge processing? JA was left-hemisphere language dominant and suffered a lesion confined to right mid- and anterior fusiform gyrus. In the presence of intact language abilities, JA had partially lost knowledge of visual attributes of biological or non-biological entities, independently of task: Object discrimination, oral feature generation, forced-choice naming-to-definition, or free-hand drawing. Functional-associative or non-visual sensory attributes were spared. The same region that was lesioned in JA was activated in an fMRI study in 27 volunteers who retrieved semantic associations between concepts but only if concepts were represented as pictures and not as words. Right fusiform gyrus critically contributes to conscious recollection of visual attributes of familiar entities.

6.2 Introduction

We mean many different things when we say we know what an entity, like "horse", is [324]. To uncover the neurobiological basis of this multifaceted knowledge is one of cognitive neuroscience's central endeavours [21] [122]. A key source of evidence are human brain lesions that impair knowledge, e.g. of specific attributes such as visual features [136] [137] [138] [139] [22] [140] or of specific categories such as biological entities [136] [113] [141] [142] [137] [138] [22] [139]. The underlying lesions are either left-sided [141] [137] [22] [140] or bi-hemispheric [136] [141] [138] [139] [140]. Most typically the knowledge deficits come to the attention because of a picture naming deficit that is category-specific [136] [141] [142] [22]. This naming impairment may be associated with category-specific impairment of comprehension [113] [141], drawing [22], picture identification [136] [22] or a category-specific deficit of knowledge about visual attributes of pictures [136] [22].

A second source of evidence about knowledge of visual attributes of concrete entities are studies of mental imagery in patients [325] [326] and in healthy volunteers [327] [328]. Deficits of mental image generation principally arise from left-sided or bi-hemispheric lesions [325]. In healthy controls, category effects during visual imagery are predominantly lateralised to the left [328]. Our first question was whether a lesion that is confined to the non-dominant hemisphere and leaves naming intact can impair knowledge of concrete entities.

Second, we determined the place of this right-hemispheric component within the organised structure of knowledge in the human brain. According to a distributed model of conceptual processing [329] [21], knowledge of visual attributes of familiar objects relies on distributed mnemonic representations that can be directly accessed from 3D structural descriptions of concrete entities [21] [330] [331] [114] [329] [332]. Structural descriptions code for long-term memory of perceptual features that are necessary for identification of familiar objects, especially shape and object parts [22] [24]. According to the Hierarchical Interactive Theory (HIT) of visual object processing [22] [24], structural descriptions also provide visuoperceptual input with an "access code" to the associative-semantic knowledge system [333]. Within the right hemisphere, we examined the neuroanatomical relationship between these 3 processes: Retrieval of knowledge of visual attributes of familiar entities, object identification and naming, and input modality-specific access to the left-hemispheric associative-semantic system.

We combined a patient lesion study with functional magnetic resonance imaging. A right ventral occipital lesion in a left-hemisphere language dominant patient caused partial loss of knowledge of visual attributes of familiar entities, regardless of task output modality, oral or by drawing. The lesion coincided with an area that was normally activated when subjects judged semantic associations between entities represented as pictures but not when entities were represented as words.

6.3 Methods

All participants gave written informed consent and the experiments were approved by the Ethical Committee, University Hospital Gasthuisberg, Leuven. Fifteen controls (mean age: 61.9 years, s.d. 5.9; years of education: 14.0, s.d. 2.2) participated in the behavioral experiments as well as patients JA and MV. Twenty-seven strictly right-handed controls (mean age: 66.5 years, s.d. 8.3, years of education: 13.5, s.d. 2.8) as well as JA participated in the fMRI experiment. All experiments were conducted using Superlab for PC version 2.0 (Cedrus).

6.3.1 Subjects

JA, a strictly right-handed 58-year old woman with 16 years of education and a history of arterial hypertension, suffered 9 months prior to presentation a unifocal ischemic stroke confined to the right mid- and anterior fusiform gyrus (Figs. 6.1*a*,*b* and 6.2*a*). The posterior half of the lesion overlapped with the Fusiform Face Area [334] (Fig. 6.1*c*). The lesion also overlapped with area LO [23] (Fig. 6.1*d*) and lay just anterior to retinotopically defined area V4v. Its posterior border was symmetrical to a left-sided area in JA that had a lower as well as an upper visual field representation, possibly area V8 [335] (Fig. 6.1*e*).

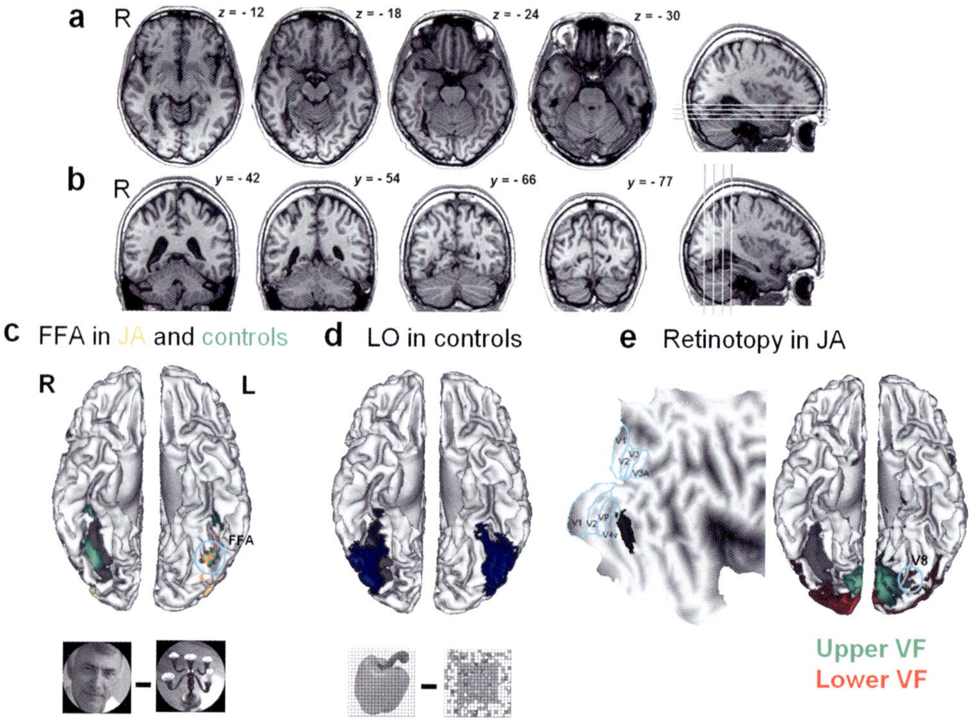

Figure 6.1: Neuroanatomy of JA's lesion. (**a,b**) T1 structural MRI in JA acquired 1 year after lesion onset. (**a**) Transverse sections. (**b**) Coronal sections. (**c**) Fusiform Face Area (FFA) localising experiment (voxel-level inference uncorrected $P \prec 0.001$). Green: Faces minus objects in 2 healthy controls; Yellow: Faces minus objects in JA. Activity maps are superposed onto JA's ventral brain surface using CARET software (Washington University School of Medicine, Department of Anatomy and Neurobiology, http://brainmap.wustl.edu). The left-sided FFA in JA and controls is encircled by the cyan line. (**d**) LO localising experiment (voxel-level inference uncorrected $P \prec 0.001$). Blue: LO in 6 healthy controls. (**e**) Flattened brain surface: JA's lesion superposed onto a standard map with standard delineation (cyan) of retinotopic areas V1 to V4v using CARET software. Ventral brain surface: Representation of upper (green) and lower (red) visual field in JA (voxel-level inference uncorrected $P \prec 0.001$). Putative area V8, an area with a representation of both upper and lower visual field, is encircled in cyan.

JA had a left upper quadrantanopia. She scored 22/24 on the Ishihara color test. Her visuoperceptual dysfunction consisted principally of impaired visuoperceptual feature matching [106], prosopagnosia, and impairment on the Object Decision [107] [106], the Silhouettes and the Progressive Silhouettes tasks [107] (table 6.1).

	JA	MV	norms mean (s.d.)	cut-off
Boston Naming Test (/60)	49	**26**	54.6 (6.1)	-
Animal Verbal Fluency	12	17	22.2 (5.1)	-
Akense Afasie test [101]				
Naming (/120)	115	**108**	117.3 (3.4)	-
Comprehension (/120)	111	**101**	113.8 (4.9)	-
Token Test (/50)	1	1	0.8 (1.5)	-
Spontaneous speech (/30)	30	30	30.0 (0.0)	-
Psycholinguistic Assesment of Language Processing in Aphasia verbal association test [103]				
High imagibility (/15)	**7**	14	14.1 (1.0)	-
Low imagibility (/15)	**12**	15	14.4 (0.9)	-
Birmingham Object Recognition Battery [106]				
Copy	nl	nl	nl	-
Length match (/30)	**17**	28	26.9 (1.6)	-
Size match (/30)	**17**	28	27.3 (2.4)	-
Orientation match (/30)	**12**	28	24.8 (2.6)	-
Position of gap match (/40)	**23**	38	35.1 (4.0)	-
Overlapping figures (mean time in s)				
Letters				
single	**32.5**	9	7.9	11.2
paired non-overlapping	**26.5**	19	13.8	22.6
paired overlapping	**53.5**	21.5	16	25.7
triplets non-overlapping	**56**	26	22.3	34.9
triplets overlapping	**96**	33.5	23.9	35.1
Geometric shapes				
single	**45.5**	23	18.4	24.4
paired non-overlapping	**67**	29.5	38.9	65.2
paired overlapping	**104**	31.5	39	65.9
triplets non-overlapping	118	44	65	133.9
triplets overlapping	**143**	69	69	136.9
Line drawings				
single	18	**54**	14	40.9
paired non-overlapping	27	**85**	21.5	49.9
paired overlapping	44	**101**	23.9	66.9
Minimal feature view match (/25)	23	25	23.3 (2.0)	-
Foreshortened view match (/25)	24	25	21.6 (2.6)	-
Object decision				
hard (/32)	**18**	28	27.3 (1.9)	-
easy (/32)	**22**	29	29.8 (1.7)	-
Item match (/32)	30	31	30	26
Association match (/32)	29	27	27.5 (2.4)	-
Naming living things (/15)	14	**2**	12.7 (2.2)	-
Visual Object and Space Perception Battery [107]				
Incomplete letters (/22)	14	19	-	16
Silhouettes (/30)	**6**	24	-	15
Object decision (/20)	**7**	18	-	14
Progressive silhouettes (/20)	16	17	-	15
Hooper (/30)	19	24	25.7 (4.7)	-
Benton facial recognition test (/54)	**36**	48	48.2 (3.7)	-
Auditory Verbal Learning Test				
Learning (/75)	55	13	49.4 (9.3)	-
Recall (/15)	14	**1**	10.9 (2.1)	-
Recognition (/15)	15	**3**	14.3 (1.3)	-
Coloured Progressive Matrices (/36)	33	32	31.2 (3.2)	-

Table 6.1: Neuropsychological profile in JA and MV. Bold: Below cut-off or $\prec$ 2 s.d. below normal mean

Controls consisted of 15 and 27 healthy age- and education-matched volunteers who participated in the behavioral and the functional magnetic resonance imaging (fMRI) study, respectively, as well as a second patient, MV (age: 71 years, 14 years of education), a man who was tested approximately one year after a purely left-sided ischemic lesion in a region roughly symmetrical to that lesioned in JA (Fig. 6.2*b* and Table 6.1).

6.3.2 Knowledge of visual attributes

In the feature generation task (Fig. 6.3*a*) a written name of a concrete entity was presented on the screen for 1 min and subjects were instructed to generate orally as many different kinds of characteristics as possible within 1 minute. We probed 5 entities per category and 11 different categories (8 biological, 3 non-biological) (Fig. 6.3*a*). Entities were selected on the basis of normative data [336] and covered a range of frequencies and typicalities [336].

Responses were recorded and the number of visual and of nonvisual sensory attributes as well as encyclopaedic, categorical and functional-associative attributes were counted. The latter 3 types were pooled for behavioral analysis. We also determined how many visual attributes that belonged to a particular type (color, size, shape, texture, motion and object parts) were generated by JA and controls (Fig. 6.3*b*).

We compared the individual patient's scores with that of control sample by means of a modified *t* test [337] (http://www.abdn.ac.uk/ psy086/dept/psychom.htm) (statistical threshold one-tailed $P \prec 0.05$). We used the following criteria [338] to define a dissociation between tests X and Y: The patient had to be significantly impaired on test X compared to controls [337] and the discrepancy between test X and test Y had to be statistically different from the discrepancy observed in controls (Revised Standardized Difference test [338]) (http://www.abdn.ac.uk/ psy086/dept/psychom.htm) (two-tailed $P \prec 0.05$).

Approximately 6 months after the feature generation task subjects were asked to draw on verbal command the same 55 concrete entities as used in the feature generation task, using a black pen. In addition, one week later JA was asked to copy a drawing of each entity, selected randomly from the controls' drawings. Drawings by controls, JA and MV were scanned as well as copies by JA of drawings by controls. Recognizability of the drawings was measured by asking 40 healthy subjects to name the drawing. Each entity was shown once per subject and the origin of the drawing (JA, controls, or copy by JA of controls' drawings) was counterbalanced across subjects. Recognizability was analysed using a one-way repeated-measures ANOVA with origin (JA, MV, controls or copies by JA of controls' drawings) as factor. Bonferroni correction was used for post-hoc comparisons.

Subjects also participated in a more constrained, forced-choice response task, the forced-choice naming-to-definition task [99] (Fig. 6.3*c*). We presented on the screen a written definition based on either visual or functional-associative attributes. Subjects had to press a key when they had read and understood the definition. This initiated the two-choice response phase: The target name and the distractor were presented to the left or to the right of the screen. The distractor belonged to the same sub-category as the target [99]. Subjects had to press a left- or right-hand key depending on the position of the matching stimulus. The definitions were based on either visual (biological: 55, non-biological: 42) or functional-associative (biological: 40, non-biological: 25) attributes and were translated from the original version of this task [99]. In total we probed 162 entities from 6 biological categories (body parts, vegetables, fruits, insects, animals or birds) and 6 non-biological categories (furniture, kitchen utensils, clothes, vehicles tools or musical instruments). Performance in patients and controls was statistically analysed as described above [337] [338].

We re-tested JA after 1 year and determined within-item, between-session (1 year interval) consistency for the forced-choice naming-to-definition task [339] [332]. We determined the proportion of consistent failures and inconsistent failures and calculated parameters for "r(etrieval)" and "s(torage)" using a 2-parameter Markov chain stochastic model [339].

6.3.3 Object identification and name retrieval

In the confrontation naming task [168] (Fig. 6.2*c,d*) subjects had to name 60 line drawings from the Snodgrass and Vanderwart set (1980) [129], covering 3 biological (10 animate, 10 fruits and 10 vegetables) and 3 non-biological categories (10 tools, 10 furniture, 10 vehicles). The stimulus set was matched between categories for frequency, visual complexity, familiarity, image agreement, and prototypicality. Responses were recorded and voice key latencies were determined digitally (Adobe Audition 1.5, Adobe Systems Incorporated).

In the speeded picture identification task (Fig. 6.2*e,f*), subjects had to name line drawings [129] of 48 exemplars from 5 biological categories (8 birds, 8 insects, 8 mammals, 12 fruits and 12 vegetables) and 48 exemplars from 5 non-biological categories (11 tools, 10 vehicles, 11 articles of furniture, 6 parts of buildings and 10 kitchen utensils). A trial consisted of a forward mask (200 ms duration), followed by a picture which was immediately followed by a backward mask (200 ms duration). Masks were scrambled pictures. Test stimulus presentation duration varied between 50, 100, 150, 300, 500, 800, 1500, and 3000 ms. Each stimulus was shown once only per subject. Subjects were instructed to name the picture. The inter-trial interval was 5000 ms. Performance of these tasks by patients and controls was statistically analysed as described above [337] [338].

6.3.4 Associative-semantic knowledge

Tasks and stimuli

The design of the fMRI experiment was factorial and similar to that of previous studies [128] [5] [174]. The first factor, task, had two levels: Associative-semantic versus visuoperceptual judgment. The second factor, input modality, also had two levels: Line drawings versus printed words. The associative semantic condition consisted of a modified version of the Pyramids and Palm Trees test [128] [5]. During a trial, a triplet of stimuli was presented for 5250 ms, one stimulus on top (the sample stimulus) and one in each lower quadrant (the test stimuli). Subjects had to press a left- or right-hand key depending on which of the two test stimuli matched the sample stimulus more closely in meaning. A given triplet was presented in either the picture or the word format and this was counterbalanced across subjects. In the visuoperceptual control condition, a stimulus was presented in three different sizes. Subjects had to press a left or right-hand key depending on which of the two test stimuli matched the sample stimulus more closely in size on the screen. Two successive trials were separated by a 1500 ms interval. Each epoch, i.e. a block of trials of the same type, consisted of 4 trials (total duration 27 s).

Stimuli were presented at 3.8 deg eccentricity. The pictures were taken from the Snodgrass-Vanderwart set [129]. Mean picture size was 5.6 deg and letter size 1.5 deg.

In the main experiment, during a trial of the associative-semantic conditions pictures or names of 3 different entities were displayed while during a trial of the visuoperceptual conditions we presented pictures or names of 1 entity in 3 different sizes. In a sensory control experiment in which 5 healthy controls participated, we presented stimuli identical to those shown in each of the 4 conditions of the main experiment while subjects performed a central target detection task. They had to press a right-hand button when the fixation point dimmed. Target frequency was 0 to 4 dimmings per 6750 ms (mean: 2, s.d. 1.3).

fMRI image acquisition and analysis

A 1.5 tesla Siemens Sonata system (Siemens Medical Solutions) equipped with an 8-channel receive-only head coil (MRI Devices Corp.) provided a T1-weighted structural volume (coronal inversion recovery prepared three-dimensional gradient echo images; Inversion time 800 ms, TE/TR 3.93/1950 ms) as well as T2* echo-planar images (EPI) (42 sagittal slices; voxel size 3x3x3 mm^3; TE/TR 40/3000 ms). A total of 116 volumes were acquired during each run. Each run consisted of 3 replications of each of the 4 conditions. Subjects underwent 4 to 6 runs each.

We used Statistical Parametric Mapping 2002. After realignment and normalisation [180] the EPI volumes were spatially smoothed using a 6 mm full-width-of-half-maximum (FWHM) isotropic Gaussian kernel. A high-pass filter of 216 sec was applied and a low-pass filter consisting of a canonical hemodynamic response function (HRF). The epoch-related response was modeled by a boxcar convolved with a canonical HRF. For each subject a t statistic for the parameter estimates was generated for the contrast between the associative-semantic and the visuoperceptual conditions for words and pictures together and also for each input-modality separately. We also tested the interaction between task and input-modality. The individuals' t maps were transformed to Z maps and entered into a second level analysis. At second level, we carried out a random-effects within-group analysis of the data obtained in controls using a one-sample t test. The significance map was thresholded at a voxel-level inference threshold of $P \prec 0.001$ and cluster-level inference of $P \prec 0.05$ corrected for the entire brain volume. An identical procedure was followed for analysis of the sensory control experiment.

We also conducted 3 localising experiments. In a first experiment we localised FFA in JA and 2 controls by means of the contrast of faces minus objects [334] (Fig. 6.1*c*). In a second localising experiment in 6 healthy controls we localised LO by means of the contrast of objects minus scrambled objects [340] [23] (Fig. 6.1*d*). In a third experiment we mapped upper and lower visual field representations in JA [28] (Fig. 6.1*e*). Stimuli were filled with flickering colored random checkerboards. JA underwent 3 runs with upper and lower visual field stimuli. Each run consisted of 120 volumes with 6 replications of each of the 2 conditions. This retinotopic experiment was carried out in a Philips Intera 3T scanner (50 axial slices; voxel size 2.75 mm^3; TE/TR 30/3000 ms).

6.4 Results

6.4.1 Knowledge of visual attributes

We probed JA's knowledge of concrete entities using tasks that did not rely on pictorial input [341] (Fig. 6.3). We provided the name of a concrete entity and instructed subjects to orally generate as many different kinds of its characteristics as possible within 1 minute. We collected data from 11 different categories (8 biological, 3 non-biological), each probed by means of 5 exemplars selected across a range of frequencies and typicalities [336] (Fig. 6.3*a*). JA generated significantly fewer visual attributes than healthy controls ($t = -3.01$, $P = 0.005$) while generation of functional-associative attributes ($t = 1.08$, $P = 0.15$) or non-visual sensory attributes ($t = -0.17$, $P = 0.43$) did not differ between JA and controls (Fig. 6.3*a*). The differ-

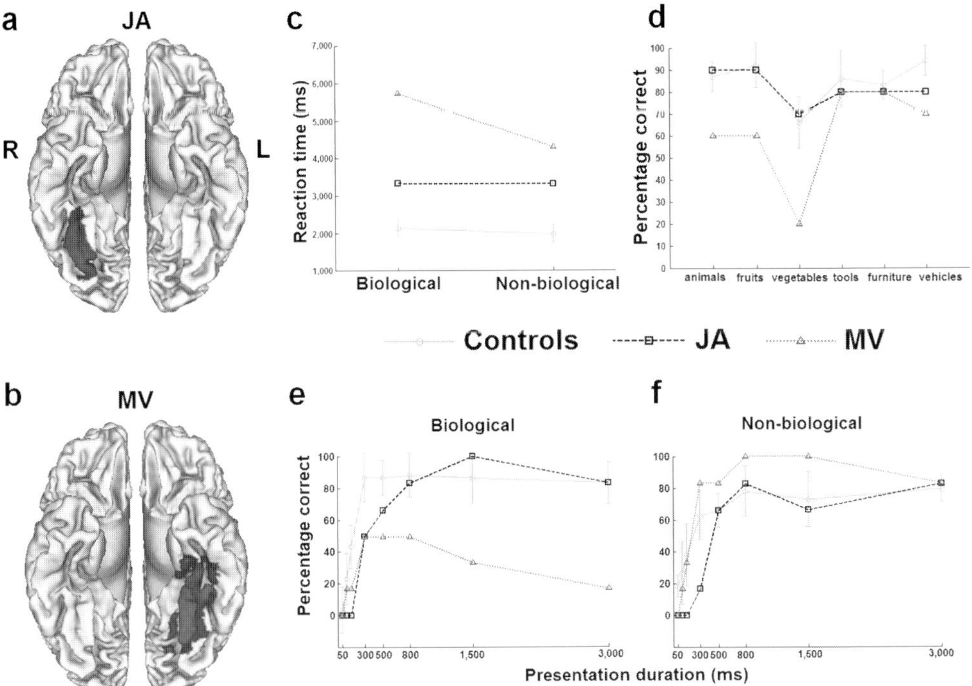

Figure 6.2: Object identification and name retrieval in JA, MV and controls. JA's lesion (**a**) and MV's lesion (**b**) projected onto the ventral brain surface. (**c,d**) Confrontation naming task. Reaction times (**c**) and accuracies (**d**) for biological and non-biological items (mean and s.d.). (**e,f**) Time-accuracy functions for speeded picture identification for biological (**e**) and non-biological (**f**) entities in JA, MV and 15 healthy matched controls. Mean and s.d. X-axis: Presentation duration in ms. Y-axis: Percentage correct.

ence between visual attributes and functional-associative attributes was significantly larger in JA than in controls ($t = -3.06$, $P = 0.008$), fulfilling criteria for a dissociation between visual and functional-associative attributes [338]. This was also the case for the difference between visual and non-visual sensory attributes ($t = -2.15$, $P = 0.049$). Among the visual attributes, JA generated significantly fewer colors ($t = -2.22$, $P = 0.022$), shapes ($t = -3.46$, $P = 0.002$), and object parts ($t = -2.063$, $P = 0.029$) than controls (Fig. 6.3*b*). There was no category effect ($t = 0.80$, two-tailed $P = 0.44$). This contrasted with the left-sided lesion patient MV who showed category-specificity without attribute-specificity. MV generated significantly fewer attributes for biological than for non-biological entities compared to controls ($t = -2.62$, $P = 0.02$), regardless of type of attribute. MV's pattern of performance met criteria for a dissociation between biological and non-biological entities [338]. In MV the difference between visual attributes and functional-associative attributes did not differ from that in controls ($t = 0.24$, $P = 0.81$) nor did the difference between visual attributes and sensory non-visual attributes ($t = 0.87$, $P = 0.40$).

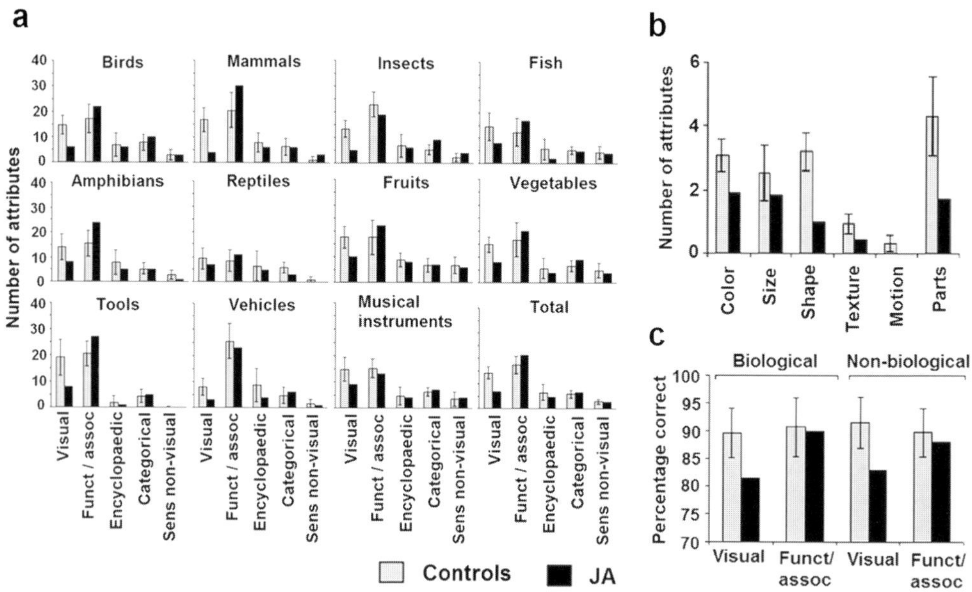

Figure 6.3: Knowledge of visual attributes. (**a,b**) Feature generation task. (**a**) For each semantic sub-category (indicated on top) and each type of attribute (indicated in the x axis (third row)), the y-axis indicates the mean number (and s.d.) of attributes generated by controls (white) and the mean number of attributes generated by JA (black). Abbreviations: Sens: Sensory; Funct/assoc: Functional-associative. The last panel titled "total" indicates the mean number of attributes generated across all sub-categories in controls and JA. (**b**) Mean number of visual attributes of a given type averaged over all 55 entities (and s.d.) generated by controls (white) and by JA (black). (**c**) Forced-choice naming-to-definition. X-axis: Type of definition: based on visual versus functional-associative attributes for biological versus non-biological entities, respectively. Y-axis: Percentage correct (mean and s.d.).

If knowledge of visual attributes is impaired, the deficit should not depend on output modality. Approximately 6 months after the feature generation task, we asked JA to draw on verbal command the same entities as those used before in the oral feature generation task. One week later, we asked her also to copy drawings from controls. JA's copies of drawings did not differ in recognizability from the original drawings she copied, thus ruling out constructional apraxia. Her drawings on verbal command however were significantly less recognizable than drawings by controls ($P \prec 0.0005$), than her copies of drawings from controls ($P \prec 0.000001$) or than drawings by MV ($P \prec 0.000001$) ($F_{3,162} = 23.0$, $P \prec 0.000001$).

If JA's deficit is partly due to a loss of knowledge of visual attributes, JA should also be impaired on a more constrained, forced-choice naming-to-definition task. When definitions of concrete entities were based on visual attributes and subjects had to select between two possible answers, JA was significantly less accurate than controls ($t = -2.48$, $P = 0.013$) but not when definitions were based on functional-associative attributes [99] ($t = -0.48$, $P = 0.32$) (Fig. 6.3*c*). In JA, the difference in accuracy for definitions based on visual attributes compared to that for definitions based on functional-associative attributes was significantly larger than in controls ($t = -2.16$, $P = 0.049$), confirming the presence of a task-independent dissociation between visual and functional-associative attributes [338] (Fig. 6.3*c*). JA's pattern of performance contrasted with MV who did not show any attribute effect ($t = 0.87$, $P = 0.40$) compared to controls. In JA or MV the naming-to-definition task did not reveal any category effect ($t = 0.29$, $P = 0.78$ and $t = -1.37$, $P = 0.19$, respectively). We tested JA on the same task 1 year later. An analysis of within-item between-session consistency yielded $r = 0.94$ and $s = 0.59$ [339], indicative of a high degree of within-item consistency.

6.4.2 Object identification and name retrieval

Knowledge of visual attributes of familiar objects was clearly impaired in JA. Two other essential functions are object identification and noun retrieval. We directly tested both processes by means of a confrontation naming test [168] (Fig. 6.2*c,d*). JA was slower than our controls ($t = 5.67$, $P \prec 0.001$) (Fig. 6.2*c*) but equally accurate ($t = -0.45$, $P = 0.66$) (Fig. 6.2*d*). There was no category effect (Fig. 6.2*c,d*). This contrasted with MV in whom the difference of reaction times ($t = 8.93$, $P \prec 0.00001$) and accuracies ($t = -2.24$, $P = 0.042$) between biological versus non-biological items was significantly larger than in controls (Fig. 6.2*c,d*), confirming the presence of a dissociation between biological and non-biological entities in MV [338].

Slowing of picture naming can arise at the level of picture identification or at the level of noun retrieval. To distinguish these two possibilities, we conducted a picture naming task where we varied stimulus presentation durations from 50 ms to 3000 ms (Fig. 6.2*e,f*). At stimulus durations of 150 or 300 ms JA named significantly less accurately than normal controls ($t = -2.64$, $P = 0.02$, and $t = -3.62$, $P = 0.003$, respectively) but if given sufficient time for picture identification JA named within the normal range (Fig. 6.2*e,f*). This indicates that slowing of picture naming in JA originated at the level of object identification rather than noun retrieval. There was no category effect (Fig. 6.2*e,f*). This contrasted with MV who named biological items less accurately than controls regardless of stimulus duration (for stimulus durations of 300, 500, 800, 1500 and 3000 ms $t = -2.34$, -3.22, -2.72, -3.20 and -4.87 respectively, $P \prec 0.05$) (Fig. 6.2*e*) while naming of non-biological entities fell within the normal range at all stimulus durations in patient MV (Fig. 6.2*f*).

6.4.3 Associative-semantic knowledge

Performance on the fMRI tasks

Behaviorally, subjects performed the associative-semantic task with words or with pictures (2797 ms, s.d. 346, and 2900 ms, s.d. 381; 86.3%, s.d. 7.4, and 83.2%, s.d. 6.8) more slowly and less accurately than the respective visuoperceptual conditions (2239 ms, s.d. 386, and 2409 ms, s.d. 345; 90.8%, s.d. 8.5, and 89.6%, s.d. 7.5). The main effect of task (reaction times: $F_{1,26} = 121.1$, $P \prec 0.00001$; accuracies $F_{1,26} = 24.4$, $P \prec 0.0001$) and modality (reaction times: $F_{1,26} = 21.9$, $P \prec 0.0001$; accuracies $F_{1,26} = 6.1$, $P \prec 0.05$) were significant. The task-by-modality interaction remained far below significance (reaction times: $F_{1,26} = 1.6$, $P = 0.22$; accuracies: ($F_{1,26} = 1.4$, $P = 0.25$).

JA's accuracy on the associative-semantic task did not differ significantly from controls for pictures (87.5%; $t = 0.621$, $P = 0.270$) or for words (91.6%; $t = 0.717$, $P = 0.240$) but she performed both tasks significantly more slowly than controls (3908 ms, $t = 2.60$, $P = 0.008$ and 3819 ms, $t = 2.90$, $P = 0.004$, respectively). In comparison to controls, JA was also significantly less accurate and slower on the visuoperceptual control condition with pictures (62.5%, $t = -3.55$, $P \prec 0.005$; 2409 ms, $t = 4.06$, $P \prec 0.001$) and with words (66.6%, $t = -2.80$, $P = 0.005$; 3872 ms, $t = 4.15$, $P \prec 0.001$).

fMRI results

In JA, we demonstrated a loss of knowledge of visual attributes in combination with a mild structural description loss. We examined whether the region lesioned in JA played a role in a third key process: Picture-specific access to associative-semantic knowledge [24].

In controls, a right-hemispheric area that overlapped with JA's lesion (Fig. 6.4*a* green) showed a significant task-by-modality interaction (45,–54,–24, $Z = 4.65$, extent (*ext.*) = 279, cluster-level corrected $P \prec 0.001$): It was significantly activated when subjects carried out an associative-semantic task with pictures compared to a visuoperceptual task with pictures but not when the same tasks were performed with words and were compared (Fig. 6.4*b*). The interaction arose from significant activation when subjects performed the associative-semantic compared to the visuoperceptual task with pictures (36,–51,–21, $Z = 4.03$, *ext.* = 52, cluster-level corrected $P \prec 0.001$) (Fig. 6.4*b*). The right fusiform gyrus was not activated when the same 2 tasks were compared with words as input (uncorrected $P \succ 0.05$) (Fig. 6.4*b*).

Performance differences could not account for the interaction effect since the difference in reaction times and accuracies between the associative-semantic and the visuoperceptual conditions was equated between words and pictures. Furthermore, right fusiform activity differences did not correlate with differences in reaction times or accuracies (uncorrected $P \succ 0.05$). Third, in a sub-group of controls ($n = 7$) in whom reaction times and accuracies were almost identical between the associative-semantic (2728 ms, s.d. 346; 86%, s.d. 3.1) and the visuoperceptual picture conditions (2756 ms, s.d. 561; 87.9%, s.d. 7.1) and between the associative semantic (2740 ms, s.d. 378; 88.6%, s.d. 3.6) and the visuoperceptual conditions with words (2654 ms, s.d. 432; 88.4%, s.d. 7.1), a highly significant task-by-modality interaction was present in the same right fusiform area (42, –48, –27, $Z = 6.91$, *ext.* 31, cluster-level $P \prec 0.001$ corrected for the whole brain search volume) as in the total group, thus ruling out performance differences as an explanation.

The right fusiform activity cluster that showed a significant task-by-modality interaction extended into the right middle occipital gyrus (48,–78, 3, $Z = 3.52$). One other area that showed higher activity during the associative-semantic condition with pictures and a significant task-by-modality interaction was the left fusiform gyrus (Fig. 6.4*a* green) (–45,–48,–21, *ext.* 43, $Z = 3.95$, cluster-level corrected $P \prec 0.005$).

In the sensory control experiment where subjects carried out a central target detection task, activity did not differ in the right fusiform gyrus between the picture conditions (Fig. 6.4*c*).

Otherwise, in the left hemisphere, an input-modality independent distributed system was activated during the associative-semantic compared to the visuoperceptual task for words as well as for pictures (Fig. 6.4*d-f*). This left-hemispheric system comprised left occipitotemporal

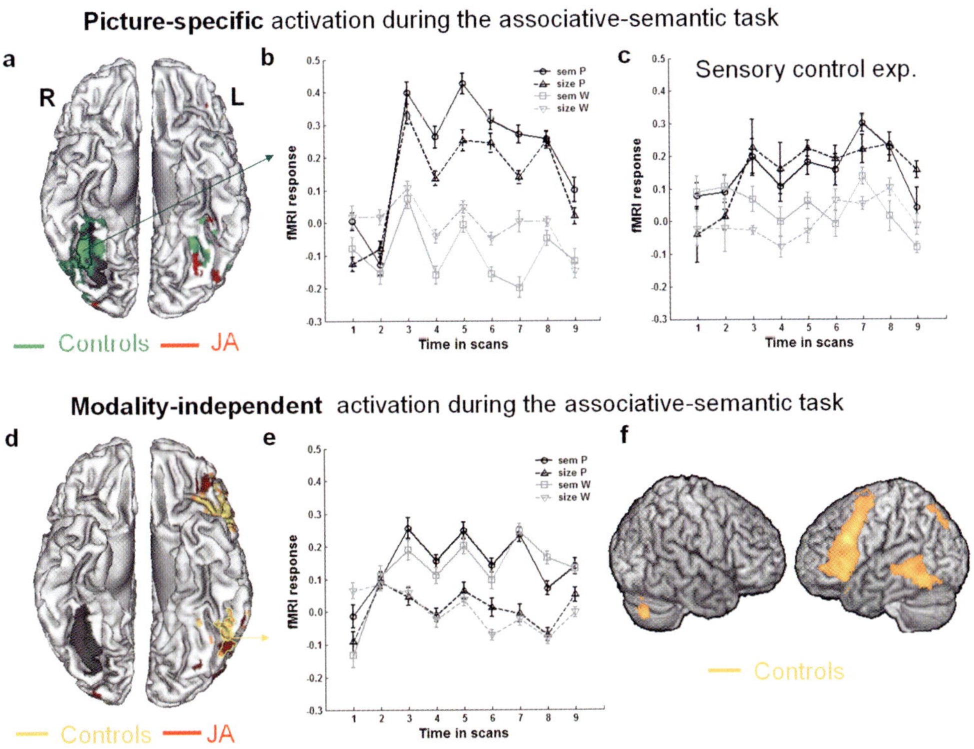

Figure 6.4: Associative-semantic knowledge. (**a,b**) Modality-by-task interaction: (Associative-semantic task with pictures – Visuoperceptual task with pictures) – (Associative-semantic task with words – visuoperceptual task with words). (**a**) Z map obtained in healthy controls (green) and in JA (red), superposed onto the ventral surface of JA's brain. Voxel-level threshold $P \prec 0.001$. Activity in voxels within the dark green boundary reaches a significance threshold of $P \prec 0.0001$ in controls. (**b**) Activity profile (mean and s.e.m.) averaged over the cluster of right fusiform voxels included within the dark green boundary shown in **a** (47 voxels) and over all 27 subjects. Abbreviations: Sem: Associative semantic task. Size: Visuoperceptual task. P: Pictures. W: Words. (**c**) Sensory control experiment (exp.). Activity profile averaged over the same voxels as those included for the profile shown in b and over all 27 subjects. (**d,e,f**) Conjunction between the contrast (Associative-semantic task with pictures – Visuoperceptual task with pictures) and the contrast (Associative-semantic task with words – visuoperceptual task with words). (**d**) Z map obtained in healthy controls (yellow) and Z map obtained in JA (red). Voxel-level threshold $P \prec 0.001$. Activity in voxels within the bright yellow boundary reaches a significance threshold of $P \prec 0.0001$ in controls. (**c**) Activity profile (mean and s.e.m.) averaged over the cluster of left inferior temporal voxels included within the bright yellow boundary shown in **d** (82 voxels) and over all 27 subjects. (**f**) Z map obtained in healthy controls (yellow) superposed onto the brain convexity.

junction, inferior and middle temporal gyrus, inferior frontal sulcus and inferior frontal gyrus, confirming previous results [5]. The input-modality independent ventral occipitotemporal activation (Fig. 6.4*d* yellow) lay lateral to the picture-specific left fusiform activation (Fig. 6.4*a* green).

JA also participated in the fMRI experiment. Her left-hemispheric activity pattern during associative-semantic processing did not differ from that seen in controls, confirming left-hemispheric dominance in JA. During associative-semantic judgements with pictures however compared to visuoperceptual judgements, she did not activate the right fusiform area, which coincided with her lesion, but she did activate the left fusiform gyrus (Fig. 6.4*a* red) and right middle occipital gyrus similarly to controls (task-by-modality interaction in JA: –45,–60,–30, *ext.* 28, $Z = 4.66$, cluster-level corrected $P \prec 0.05$ and 45,–90,6, *ext.* 40, $Z = 4.51$, cluster-level corrected $P \prec 0.005$).

6.5 Discussion

Previous functional imaging studies in healthy controls have revealed bilateral ventral occipitotemporal activation during knowledge retrieval tasks [342] [328]. Our study revealed what is a critical contribution of the right-sided fusiform gyrus to knowledge processing (Fig. 6.3). When lesioned, the impact of right fusiform dysfunction upon retrieval of visual attributes cannot be fully compensated for by the intact left fusiform gyrus or by more anterior temporal areas (Fig. 6.3). Our patient data provide strong evidence that processes in the right mid- and anterior fusiform gyrus are critically important for full conscious recollection of visual attributes of familiar objects [343]. Already at this level, the vision system is not encapsulated [344] but is consciously accessible and contributes to cognitive processing [345] [341]. JA's pattern of impairment could be accounted for by a blurring of the mental image she has of concrete objects [327] [325] [326] [346]. Detailed knowledge of how an object looks like is required for drawing on verbal command, for distinguishing real and pseudo-objects, for conscious generation of visual features of named objects as well as for naming to verbal definitions based on visual attributes [325]. Our data provide strong evidence in favor of a right-hemispheric system that mediates conscious recollection of visual attributes of familiar concrete entities.

To our knowledge, only in left-hemispheric (GG and AV [137], SRB [22], IOC [140]) or bihemispheric lesion patients (Michelangelo [136], KR [142], DM [138], EC [139], PCO [140]) has selective impairment of knowledge of visual [140] cortical dysfunction was relatively diffuse, Michelangelo [136], GG and AV [137] had large temporal lesions due to Herpes simplex encephalitis and SRB [22] had suffered a large occipitotemporal hemorrhagic stroke. In one patient, IOC [140], who had a left posterior cerebral artery stroke, object color knowledge retrieval was selectively impaired with preservation of knowledge of other visual attributes. Similarly to JA, patients DM [138], Michelangelo [136], GG and AV [137], SRB [22], EC [139], and PCO [140] had structural description loss. The latter six were also tested on drawing on command and were impaired in the absence of constructional apraxia, like JA. In contrast with JA, each of the cited cases had picture naming deficits which were often severe [136] [138] [137] [22] [139]. Michelangelo [136], KR [142], DM [138], GG [137], SRB [22] and EC [139] also showed category-specific effects, with biological entities more impaired than non-biological. This contrasts with JA in whom naming was accurate and semantic category had no significant effect (Fig. 6.2). JA was therefore unique in demonstrating the critical contribution of the non-language dominant right hemisphere to visual knowledge processing. Knowledge deficits in cases such as JA may remain unheeded because of the intact language capabilities. Her visual knowledge deficit was not an all-or-none phenomenon but a relative deficit. In JA memory of visual attributes that are needed for picture identification (shape, object parts) was sufficient to support accurate naming if there were no time constraints (Fig. 6.2*d-f*). JA was still able to generate visual attributes and to carry out the forced-choice naming-to-definition task based on visual attributes, but at a performance level below that observed in controls (Fig. 6.3*a,b,d*). This fits with a distributed model of visual knowledge processing. Integrity of the right fusiform gyrus is required for full and detailed visual knowledge retrieval but other areas which were intact, such as JA's homotopical fusiform region in the left hemisphere, also support visual knowledge processing and may explain why tasks such as time-unconstrained object naming appeared relatively intact.

The right mid- and anterior fusiform region was activated when healthy controls judged associative semantic relations between concrete entities and these entities were represented as pictures but not as words (Fig. 6.4*a,b*). When pictures rather than words are used as input modality for associative-semantic matching, the task solving strategy may be biased towards retrieval of semantic associations afforded by visual properties. Alternatively, within the framework of HIT the overlap between the task-by-modality interaction and the lesion may indicate that the structural description system provided pictures with an "access code" to the left-hemispheric system for associative-semantic knowledge [22]. Despite her lesion, JA performed the associative-semantic task with words or pictures accurately. This dissociation between structural description loss and associative-semantic matching has been described before (e.g. SRB) [22] [24]. A correct solution of the Pyramids and Palm Trees [128] task may be possible even when the patient is unable to retrieve in detail all visual attributes of the objects represented. Furthermore, other areas that showed a group-by-task interaction in controls as well as JA, such as left fusiform (Fig. 6.4*a*) and right middle occipital gyrus, may be able to compensate for the loss of right fusiform access to associative-semantic knowledge.

The patient lesion and the neuroimaging findings constitute converging evidence that the fusiform gyrus of the non-language dominant hemisphere is critically important for conscious recollection of visual attributes ranging from shape and object parts to color (Fig. 6.3*a,c*). The same region is involved in retrieval of associative-semantic knowledge from pictures but not from words as input (Fig. 6.4*a*). Specificity for visual attributes and for non-verbal visual input as well as a non-verbal format of representation are 3 defining characteristics of what has been termed a visual semantics system [347] [329] [348] [115]. Our data constitute converging evidence that a critical component of the visual semantics system thus defined lies within the right mid-fusiform gyrus.

To conclude, the fusiform gyrus of the non-dominant hemisphere (Fig. 6.1) contributes in a critical way to knowledge about visual attributes of familiar objects (Fig. 6.3). Our findings establish the neurobiological validity of a non-verbal right-hemispheric system for knowledge of visual attributes of concrete entities.

Chapter 7

Summary and conclusion

In this thesis, we describe the functional contribution of different brain areas to language and knowledge processes and we shed light on disease mechanisms underlying cognitive dysfunction in patients with neurodegenerative disorders.

Chapter 2

In chapter 2, we examined the neural substrate of language impairment in PPA cross-sectionally. We tested the hypothesis that, similar to aphasia due to stroke, language-related activity would shift towards right-sided areas homotopical to left-sided areas hit by the disease. Nineteen PPA patients participated, 19 healthy subjects and 14 patients with amnestic mild cognitive impairment who served as controls. A factor analysis of the neuropsychological data isolated 4 factors, with a cluster of language tests explaining the largest amount of total variance. We entered the individual factor scores as regressors into a regression analysis. Outcome variables were brain volume and response amplitude during the associative-semantic versus control conditions. Language competence correlated *positively* with volume and with responses in left anterior temporal cortex but *inversely* with responses in the right-sided homotope. In normals, anterior temporal activation was more extensive to the left than the right (laterality index (LI) 0.64 (s.e. +0.11). Laterality was inverted in PPA with word comprehension deficit (LI -0.34, s.e. 0.19), with an intermediate pattern in PPA without comprehension deficit (LI 0.23 (s.e. +0.14)). We showed a rightward laterality shift in PPA, similar to previous reports in aphasic stroke.

Chapter 3

In chapter 3, we studied the cognitive basis of impaired word retrieval in PPA across languages. We studied 12 patients with PPA of which 6 were English-speaking and 6 were Dutch-speaking. We included one normal control group consisting of 15 age-matched cognitively intact subjects as well as two disease control groups consisting of 7 patients with early-stage clinically probable Alzheimer's disease (PRAD) and 5 with mild cognitive impairment (MCI). Subjects had to name a picture (the probe) which was preceded by a written word (the prime) that could be the correct name of the picture, a noun belonging to the same semantic subcategory (related prime), a semantically unrelated noun (unrelated prime), or a pseudoword (neutral control).

Naming latencies were longer in PPA and PRAD than in controls. Critically, the interaction between group and prime type was highly significant. PPA patients named the probe more slowly following a related compared to an unrelated prime. In contrast, PRAD and MCI patients and normal controls tended to name the probe faster when preceded by a related prime. The semantic interference effect in PPA generalised across languages, English or Dutch, and PPA subtypes, fluent or non-fluent. Selection among competing word-forms sharing a same semantic field was abnormal in PPA.

Chapter 4

In chapter 4, we identified neural predictors and correlates of naming decline in PPA longitudinally. We included eighteen PPA patients and 15 healthy subjects. To identify neural predictors of naming decline, we compared gray matter volume at time of inclusion between PPA patients who declined in a one-year period and patients who did not. To study the neural substrate of progression of naming impairment, we correlated change of naming performance with change of gray matter volume. The degree of left anterior temporal atrophy was predictive of the rate of naming decline. Naming decline was associated with decreases in left posterior inferior temporal and right-sided temporal gray matter volume.

Chapter 5

In chapter 5, we examined whether the brain system for associative-semantic judgements with words or with pictures is affected in amnestic mild cognitive impairment (MCI), a prodromal stage of Alzheimer's disease, and how this relates to off-line chronometric analysis of word reading and picture naming. A consecutive memory-clinic based series of 13 amnestic MCI patients participated as well as 13 matched controls. One area, the lower bank of the posterior third of the left superior temporal sulcus (STS), showed a significant group-by-task interaction: In controls, it was activated during the associative-semantic condition with words compared to the visuoperceptual control condition but not when the same tasks were compared with pictures as input. In MCI, this word-specific activation was significantly reduced. Response amplitude correlated with subclinical word identification problems. Our data provided converging evidence for a critical contribution of the lower bank of the left posterior STS to mapping word form onto word meaning (lexical-semantic retrieval).

Chapter 6

In chapter 6, we determined the critical contribution of the right hemisphere to knowledge processing. JA was left-hemisphere language dominant and suffered a lesion confined to right mid- and anterior fusiform gyrus. In the presence of intact language abilities, JA had partially lost knowledge of visual attributes of biological or non-biological entities, independently of task: Object discrimination, oral feature generation, forced-choice naming-to-definition, or free-hand drawing. Functional-associative or non-visual sensory attributes were spared. The same region that was lesioned in JA was activated in 27 volunteers who retrieved semantic associations between concepts but only if concepts were represented as pictures and not as words. We established the critical contribution of the right fusiform gyrus to conscious recollection of visual attributes of familiar entities.

Conclusion

In 2002, we started from a model of functional anatomy of language and semantic memory in normals and tested this model in patients. The insights provided by this project allowed us to modify the model substantially.

According to our experimental model, picture-specific access to the semantic system is mediated via the left posterior inferior temporal sulcus [5]. Our data indicate that the right mid-fusiform gyrus and middle occipital gyrus contribute to this function [286]: This region is activated during associative-semantic compared to visuoperceptual tasks with pictures but not with words (Fig. 6.4*A*,*B*). Higher sensitivity of our fMRI experiment and a larger sample size (see introduction) may explain this discrepancy with our original PET findings. Dysfunction of the right fusiform gyrus leads to impaired identification of visually presented objects (Fig. 6.2) and a deficit of conscious recollection of visual attributes of concrete entities (Fig. 6.3). Specificity for visual attributes and for non-verbal visual input as well as a non-verbal format of representation are 3 defining characteristics of what has been termed a visual semantics system [329] [347] [348] [115].

Our data also indicate that the left posterior temporal cortex contains two functionally distinct but juxtaposed areas (Fig. 5.3*B*): The middle temporal gyrus which is activated during associative judgements regardless of input-modality, words or pictures, and the posterior third of the left superior temporal sulcus which is word-specific [285]. The superior temporal sulcus is activated during associative-semantic compared to visuoperceptual tasks with words but not with pictures (Fig. 5.3*A*,*C*). Dysfunction of the superior temporal sulcus leads to impaired identification of printed words at brief stimulus durations (Figs. 5.2*C* and 5.4*A*) [285].

In our a priori model, we propose that the anterior temporal poles function as associative structures that bind together representations of meaning that are distributed over human cerebral cortex [5] [241]. We demonstrate that anterior temporal atrophy or activity during associative semantic judgements with words and pictures correlates with the degree of impairment on single word processing tasks [174] [349] (Figs. 2.1 and 4.2 *A*,*C*).

We originally proposed that the left posterior inferior temporal gyrus links a visually presented object to the internal representation of its name [25] [26] [16] . Our data and other patient studies [289] [290] corroborate this view: Pathological changes of the left posterior inferior temporal gyrus leads to deterioration of picture naming performance [349] (Fig. 4.2*B*).

This project provides new insights into mechanisms of neurodegenerative disease.

We provide evidence for similar mechanism of neuronal adaptation in neurodegenerative disorders as in stroke. Recruitment of the un-affected non-dominant hemisphere is a robust finding in studies of the language system after stroke [200] [201] [202] [203]. We demonstrate that PPA, a language based neurodegenerative disorder, is also associated with a shift of activity during associative-semantic judgments towards right-hemispheric areas homotopic to the left-sided areas hit by the disease [174] (Fig. 2.1). Our project also provides clues about the cognitive architecture underlying word-finding difficulties in PPA by showing that selection among competing word forms during word retrieval is abnormal [350]. Finally, we show that a higher degree of temporal atrophy in PPA predicts a less favorable cognitive outcome within one year [349] and reveal how atrophy associated with naming impairment progresses from anterior to posterior along the inferior temporal gyrus and from left to right.

We show that amnestic MCI, a prodromal stage of Alzheimer's disease [8] [59], is associated with sub-clinical language impairment [285]. The earliest alterations of the language system are at the lexical-semantic level and involve the posterior temporal cortex. In MCI, functional imaging studies of other cognitive domains than episodic memory may also reveal which patients are at risk to convert to AD during follow-up (Figs. 5.2*B,C* and 5.4*A*).

To conclude, our approach has deepened our understanding of the functional anatomy of language and semantic memory and has provided insights into the pathogenesis of cognitive deterioration in neurodegenerative disorders.

Our findings have also opened up new avenues of research. By combining fMRI and behavioral studies in patients, we defined the different *anatomical components* of the associative-semantic system and their *functional contribution*. Insight in the *time course* of language processing and the *connectivity* among different components of the language system would complement our data.

fMRI offers excellent spatial resolution but the temporal resolution is poor. By contrast, electrophysiological methods measure neural activity directly and provide essentially unlimited temporal resolution, but suffer from low spatial resolution [351]. In the light of the complementary strengths and weaknesses of haemodynamic and electrophysiological studies, the integration of both methods will allow us to study the loci and time course of the neural activity engaged by language processes conjointly.

Measures of functional integration, such as psychophysiological interactions (PPI) [352] and dynamic causal modeling (DCM) [353] examine how interactions among brain regions are modulated by experimental manipulations. Our functional anatomical model of language will allow us to build and test a hypothetical model of effective connectivity among the different constituents.

Our study of patients at the behavioral, structural and functional anatomical level is a first step towards a more complete understanding of the disease mechanisms underlying changes of human communication. Future studies will need to establish the link between our findings and changes at more basic levels including the neurotransmitter [354], neuropathological [355] and genetic level [52] [356]. In neurodegenerative disorders, recent advances in neuroimaging [357], genetic breakthroughs [52] [53] and insights from clinicopathological correlations [47] [48] have opened a new era of translational research. Ultimately, the integrated study of behaviour, distributed brain systems, neurotransmitter systems and underlying genetic and molecular processes will lead to innovative interventional strategies.

Chapter 8

Samenvatting

Wanneer we de betekenis van woorden of figuren met elkaar vergelijken, activeren we een verspreid voornamelijk linkszijdig hersensysteem [5]. In dit project onderzochten we de functionele betekenis van de verschillende componenten van dit hersensysteem. We gebruikten hiervoor een combinatie van psychofysische en functionele anatomische studies bij normale oudere vrijwilligers en bij patiënten met corticale dysfunctie van het taalsysteem. Corticale dysfunctie was een gevolg van vasculaire corticale letsels, lichte cognitieve aantasting (mild cognitive impairment (MCI)) of primaire progressieve afasie (PPA).

We gebruikten een functioneel beeldvormingsexperiment (functionele kernspintomografie) met een factoriële design om het semantisch systeem in kaart te brengen [5]. De eerste factor, taak, bestond uit 2 niveaus: Associatief-semantisch versus visuoperceptuele beoordelingen. De tweede factor, modaliteit, bestond ook uit twee niveaus: Figuren versus woorden. De associatief-semantische taak was een aangepaste versie van de Pyramids and Palm Trees test, een klassieke neuropsychologische test [128] [32] [80]. De stimuli werden tijdens het scannen op een scherm geprojecteerd. Tijdens de actieve taak, zagen de deelnemers telkens 3 verschillende woorden of figuren, één boven, één links onder en één rechts onder. De deelnemers moesten beslissen welke van de twee onderste stimuli qua betekenis best bij de bovenste stimulus paste door links of rechts op een knop te drukken. Tijdens de visuoperceptuele controletaak zagen de deelnemers 3 keer hetzelfde woord of dezelfde figuur maar met verschillende grootte. Deelnemers moesten dan beslissen welke van de twee onderste stimuli qua grootte best bij de bovenste stimulus paste.

Normale oudere vrijwilligers activeerden een linkszijdig hersensysteem tijdens de associatief-semantische taak ten opzichte van de visuoperceptuele taak onafhankelijk van de aangeboden modaliteit, woorden of figuren. Dit hersensysteem bestond uit de gyrus frontalis inferior, de sulcus frontalis inferior en de premotorische cortex, de gyrus temporalis medius, de gyrus temporalis inferior, de occipitotemporale junctie, het middenste gedeelte van de linker fusiforme gyrus en de rechterhelft van het cerebellum. De rechter fusiforme gyrus was actief tijdens de associatief-semantische taak ten opzichte van een visuoperceptuele controletaak met figuren maar niet met woorden [286]. Omgekeerd waren de linker sulcus temporalis inferior en de linker sulcus frontalis inferior actief tijdens de associatief-semantische taak ten opzichte van een visuoperceptuele controletaak met woorden maar niet met figuren [285].

De activatie van de rechter fusiforme gyrus tijdens de associatief-semantische taak met

figuren overlapte met een corticaal letsel ten gevolge van een beroerte bij een 58-jarige patiënt. Door een gedetailleerde gedragsstudie en beeldvomingsstudie bij deze patiënt, toonden we aan dat de rechter fusiforme gyrus een kritische rol speelt bij identificatie van visueel gepresenteerde objecten en bij het oproepen van visuele kenmerken van concrete zaken, onafhankelijk van de output, verbaal of door middel van tekeningen. Specificiteit voor visuele attributen en voor niet-verbale visuele presentatie alsook een niet-verbaal formaat van representatie zijn 3 kenmerken van wat men een visueel semantisch systeem noemt [329] [347] [348] [115]. Uit onze data blijkt dat een kritische component van het visueel semantisch systeem zich in de rechter hemisfeer bevindt, meer bepaald in de rechter fusiforme gyrus.

Uit een vergelijkende studie tussen patiënten met lichte cognitieve aantasting en normale oudere vrijwilligers met overeenkomstige demografische kenmerken, bleek dat patiënten met lichte cognitieve aantasting minder activiteit vertoonden van de linker sulcus temporalis superior (STS) tijdens de associatief semantische taak [285]. Dit verschil in activiteit tussen patiënten met MCI en normalen was significant voor ***woorden*** maar niet voor figuren. Deze hypoactieve regio overlapte met de woord-specifieke associatief semantische STS regio bij normalen. In een bijkomend psychofysisch experiment, waarbij we woorden en figuren aanboden met verschillende presentatieduur, toonden we aan dat patiënten met MCI meer tijd nodig hadden dan normalen om maximum performantie te bereiken bij de idenficatie van woorden maar niet bij figuren. Daarenboven correleerde deze parameter van woord-identificatie met de activiteit in de linker STS. Deze bevindingen tonen aan dat de linker STS een kritische rol speelt bij het linken van een woord vorm aan de betekenis van dit woord en dat patiënten met lichte cognitieve aantasting een modaliteit-specifieke aantasting van het taalsysteem vertonen in tegenstelling tot patiënten met de ziekte van Alzheimer [77] [78] [79] [80] [81].

Bij patiënten met primaire progressieve afasie correleerde de ernst van de taalaantasting met de graad van atrofie en de hersenactiviteit van de linker anterieur temporale pool tijdens de associatief semantische taak, ***onafhankelijk van de modaliteit***. We vonden een omgekeerde correlatie ter hoogte van de rechter anterieur temporale pool: Hoe hoger de activiteit van de rechter anterieure gyrus temporalis medius, hoe ernstiger de aantasting van de taal. Vooral PPA patiënten met een aantasting van woordbegrip vertoonden een shift van activiteit tijdens de associatieve semantische taak van links naar rechts, zoals eerder beschreven bij patiënten na een beroerte [195] [196] [197] [198] [199] [200] [201] [202] [203]. Deze gegevens bevestigen de functie van de anterieure temporale polen als associatieve kennisstructuren en tonen, voor het eerst bij neurodegeneratieve aandoeningen, een shift van de linker taal-dominante hemisfeer naar rechts.

In een longitudinale studie van patiënten met primaire progressieve afasie toonden we aan dat de achteruitgang van de performantie op de benoemingstaak correleerde met het verlies aan grijze stof van de linker gyrus temporalis inferior en rechter temporale corticale regio's. De linker gyrus temporalis inferior overlapte met een modaliteitsonafhankelijke associatief-semantische regio geactiveerd bij normalen maar niet bij PPA. Hiermee onderschrijven we meerdere patiënten- [25] [289] [290] en beeldvormingsstudies [291] [292] [145] [293] die reeds wezen op de kritische rol van de linker posterieure gyrus temporalis inferior bij linken van visuele representaties van objecten aan hun overeenkomstige naam. Daarnaast beschreven we het anatomisch substraat van progressie van taalaantasting bij PPA.

Dit project heeft bijgedragen tot een betere kennis van de functionele betekenis van de verschillende anatomische componenten van het taalsysteem. Daarnaast hebben we bijgedragen tot een beter inzicht in de ziekte-mechanismen die gepaard gaan met cognitieve veranderingen bij neurodegeneratieve aandoeningen.

Bibliography

[1] A. Hillis. *The handbook of adult language disorders*. Psychology Press, New York, NY, 2002.

[2] P. McKenna and E.K. Warrington. Language and aphasia. In Berndt, editor, *Handbook of neuropsychology*, volume 3. Elsevier Science, Amsterdam, 2000.

[3] A.R. Damasio, D. Tranel, and M. Rizzo. Disorders of complex visual processing. In M.M. Mesulam, editor, *Principles of behavioral and cognitive neurology*, pages 332–372. Oxford University Press, New York, NY, 2000.

[4] C.J. Price, J. Crinion, and K. Friston. Design and analysis of fmri studies with neurologically impaired patients. *J Magn Reson Imaging*, 23:816–826, 2006.

[5] R. Vandenberghe, C. Price, R. Wise, O. Josephs, and R.S.J. Frackowiak. Functional anatomy of a common semantic system for words and pictures. *Nature*, 383:254–256, 1996.

[6] M.M. Mesulam. Primary progressive aphasia. *Ann Neurol*, 49:425–432, 2001.

[7] D. Neary, D.S. Snowden, L. Gustafson, U. Passant, D. Stuss, S. Black, M. Freedman, A. Kertesz, P.H. Robert, M. Albert, K. Boone, B.L. Miller, J. Cummings, and D.F. Benson. Frontotemporal lobar degeneration: a consensus on clinical diagnostic criteria. *Neurology*, 51:1546–1554, 1998.

[8] R.C. Petersen, G.E. Smith, S.C. Waring, R.J. Ivnik, E.G. Tangalos, and E. Kokmen. Mild cognitive impairment: Clinical characterization and outcome. *Arch Neurol*, 56:303–308, 1999.

[9] P. Broca. Remarques sur le sige de la facult du language articul, suivies d'une observation aphmie (pert de la parole). *Bulletin Socit Anatomique de Paris*, 36:330–357, 1861.

[10] C. Wernicke. *Der aphasische symptomencomplex*. Cohn and Weigert, Breslau, 1874.

[11] R.J.S. Wise, S.K. Scott, S.C. Blank, C.J. Mummery, K. Murphy, and E.A. Warburton. Separate neural subsystems within "Wernicke's area". *Brain*, 124:83–95, 2001.

[12] R. De Bleser. Neuroanatomy of the classical syndromes of aphasia. In R.S. Berndt, editor, *Handbook of Neuropsychology*, volume 3, pages 3–18. Elsevier Science, Amsterdam, 2001.

[13] N. Dronkers and J. Larsen. Neuroanatomy of the classical syndromes of aphasia. In R.S. Berndt, editor, *Handbook of Neuropsychology*, volume 3, pages 3–18. Elsevier Science, Amsterdam, 2001.

[14] C.J. Price. The anatomy of language: Contributions from functional neuroimaging. *J Anat*, 197:335–359, 2000.

[15] D. Howard, K. Patterson, R. Wise, W. Brown, K. Friston, C. Weiller, and R.S.J. Frackowiak. The cortical localization of the lexicons: positron emission tomography evidence. *Brain*, 115:1769–1782, 1992.

[16] C.J. Moore and C.J. Price. A functional neuroimaging study of the variables that generate category-specific object processing differences. *Brain*, 122:943–962, 1999.

[17] J.-F. Demonet, F. Chollet, S. Ramsay, D. Cardebat, J. Nespoulous, R. Wise, A. Rascol, and R. Frackowiak. The anatomy of phonological and semantic processing in normal subjects. *Brain*, 115:1753–1768, 1992.

[18] H. Damasio, T. Grabowski, D. Tranel, R. Hichwa, and A. Damasio. A neural basis for lexical retrieval. *Nature*, 380:499–505, 1996.

[19] M.T. Menard, S.M. Kosslyn, W.L. Thompson, N.M. Alpert, and S.L. Rauch. Encoding words and pictures: a positron emission tomography study. *Neuropsychologia*, 34:185–194, 1996.

[20] A.C. Nobre, T. Allison, and G. McCarthy. Word recognition in the human inferior temporal lobe. *Nature*, 372:260–263, 1994.

[21] E.M. Saffran and A. Sholl. Clues to the functional and neural architecture of word meaning. In C.M. Brown and P. Hagoort, editors, *The neurocognition of language*, pages 241–272. Oxford University Press, Oxford, 1999.

[22] E.M.E. Forde, D. Francis, M.J. Riddoch, and R.I. Rumiati. On the links between visual knowledge and naming: a single case study of a patient with a category-specific impairment for living things. *Cognitive Neuropsychology*, 14:403–458, 1997.

[23] Z. Kourtzi and N. Kanwisher. Representation of perceived object shape by the human lateral occipital complex. *Science*, 293:1506–1509, 2001.

[24] G.W. Humphreys and E.M.E. Forde. Hierarchies, similarity, and interactivity in object recognition. *Behav Brain Sci*, 24:453–+, 2001.

[25] E. De Renzi, A. Zambolin, and G. Crisi. The pattern of neuropsychological impairment associated with left posterior cerebral artery infarcts. *Brain*, 110:1099–1116, 1987.

[26] C.J. Price, C.J. Moore, G.W. Humphreys, R.S.J. Frackiowak, and K.J. Friston. The neural regions systaining object recognition and naming. *Proceedings of the Royal Society, Series B*, 263:1501–1507, 1996.

[27] R. Malach, J.B. Reppas, R.R. Benson, K.K. Kwong, H. Jiang, W.A. Kennedy, P.J. Ledden, T.J. Brady, B.R. Rosen, and R.B.H. Tootell. Object-related activity revealed by functional magnetic resonance imaging in human occipital cortex. *Proc Natl Acad Sci*, 92:8135–8139, 1995.

[28] W. Vanduffel, D. Fize, H. Peuskens, K. Denys, S. Sunaert, J.T. Todd, and G.A. Orban. Extracting 3d from motion: differences in human and monkey intraparietal cortex. *Science*, 298:413–415, 2002.

[29] E. Salmon, M. VanderLinden, F. Collette, G. Delfiore, P. Maquet, C. Degueldre, A. Luxen, and G. Franck. Regional brain activity during working memory tasks. *Brain*, 119:1617–1625, 1996.

[30] M. VanderLinden, F. Collette, E. Salmon, G. Delfiore, C. Degueldre, A. Luxen, and G. Franck. The neural correlates of updating information in verbal working memory. *Memory*, 7:549–560, 1999.

[31] M.M. Mesulam. Slowly progressive aphasia without generalized dementia. *Ann Neurol*, 11:592–598, 1982.

[32] J.R. Hodges, K. Patterson, S. Oxbury, and E. Funnell. Semantic dementia: Progressive fluent aphasia with temporal lobe atrophy. *Brain*, 115:1783–1806, 1992.

[33] J.R. Hodges and K. Patterson. Nonfluent progressive aphasia and semantic dementia: A comparative neuropsychological study. *J Internat Neuropsychol Soc*, 2:511–524, 1996.

[34] A. Kertesz, W. Davidson, P. McCabe, K. Takagi, and D. Munoz. Primary progressive aphasia: diagnosis, varieties, evolution. *J Int Neuropsychol Soc*, 9:710–719, 2003.

[35] M.M. Mesulam. Current concepts: Primary progressive aphasia: A language-based dementia. *New England Journal of Medicine*, 349:1535–1542, 2003.

[36] A. Adlam, K. Patterson, T. Rogers, P. Nestor, C. Salmond, J. Acosta-Cabronero, and J. Hodges. Semantic dementia and fluent progressive aphasia: Two sides of the same coin? *Brain*, 129:3066–3080, 2006.

[37] E. Broussolle, S. Bakchine, M. Tommasi, B. Laurent, B. Bazin, L. Cinotti, L. Cohen, and G. Chazot. Slowly progressive anarthria with late anterior opercular syndrome: a variant form of frontal cortical atrophy syndromes. *J Neurol Sci*, 144:44–58, 1996.

[38] M.L. Gorno-Tempini, N.F. Dronkers, K.P. Rankin, J.M. Ogar, L. Phengrasamy, H.J. Rosen, J.K. Johnson, M.W. Weinner, and B.L. Miller. Cognition and anatomy in three variants of primary progressive aphasia. *Ann Neurol*, 55:335–346, 2004.

[39] E. Salmon, B. Sadzot, P. Maquet, D. Dive, and G. Franck. Slowly progressive aphasia syndrome. a positron emission tomographic study. *Acta Neurol Belg*, 89:242–245, 1989.

[40] R. Sinnatamby, N.A. Antoun, C.E.L. Freer, K.A. Miles, and J.R. Hodges. Neuroradiological findings in primary progressive aphasia: CT, MRI and cerebral perfusion SPECT. *Neuroradiology*, 38:232–238, 1996.

[41] C.J. Mummery, K. Patterson, C.J. Price, J. Ashburner, R.S.J. Frackowiak, and J.R. Hodges. A voxel-based morphometry study of semantic dementia: Relationship between temporal lobe atrophy and semantic memory. *Ann Neurol*, 47:36–45, 2000.

[42] C.J. Galton, K. Patterson, K. Graham, M.A. Lambon-Ralph, G. Williams, N. Antoun, B.J. Sahakian, and J.R. Hodges. Differing patterns of temporal atrophy in Alzheimer's disease and semantic dementia. *Neurology*, 57:216–225, 2001.

[43] M.M. Mesulam, M. Grossman, A.E. Hillis, A. Kertesz, and S. Weintraub. The core and halo of primary progressive aphasia and semantic dementia. *Ann Neurol*, 54S5:S11–S14, 2003.

[44] M. Grossman, C. McMillan, P. Moore, L. Ding, G. Glosser, M. Work, and J. Gee. What's in a name: voxel-based morphometric analyses of mri and naming difficulty in Alzheimer's disease, frontotemporal dementia and corticobasal degeneration. *Brain*, 127:628–649, 2004.

[45] S.P. Sonty, M.M. Mesulam, C.K. Thompson, N.A. Johnson, S. Weintraub, T.B. Parrish, and D.R. Gitelman. Primary progressive aphasia: PPA and the language network. *Ann Neurol*, 53:35–49, 2003.

[46] J.R. Hodges, R.R. Davies, J.H. Xuereb, B. Casey, M. Broe, T.H. Bak, J.J. Kril, and G.M. Halliday. Clinicopathological correlates in frontotemporal dementia. *Ann Neurol*, 56:399–406, 2004.

[47] R.R. Davies, J.R. Hodges, J.J. Krilk, G.M. Halliday, and J.H. Xuereb. The pathological basis of semantic dementia. *Brain*, 128:1984–1995, 2005.

[48] A. Kertesz, P. McMonagle, M. Blair, W. Davidson, and D.G. Munoz. The evolution and pathology of frontotemporal dementia. *Brain*, 128:1996–2005, 2005.

[49] J.A. Knibb, J.H. Xuereb, K. Patterson, and J.R. Hodges. Clinical and pathological characterization of progressive aphasia. *Brain*, 128:1984–1995, 2005.

[50] M. Hutton, C. Lendon, P. Rizzu, M. Baker, S. Froelich, H. Houlden, S. Pickering-Brown, S. Chakraverty, A. Isaacs, A. Grover, J. Hackett, J. Adamson, S. Lincoln, D. Dickson, P. Davies, R. Petersen, M. Stevens, E. de Graaff, E. Wauters, J. van Baren, M. Hillebrand, M. Joosse, J.M. Kwon, P. Nowotny, L.K. Che, J. Norton, J. Morris, L. Reed, J. Trojanowski, H. Basun, L. Lannfelt, M. Neystat, S. Fahn, F. Dark, T. Tannenberg, P.R. Dodd, N. Hayward, J. Kwok, P. Schofield, A. Andreadis, J. Snowden, D. Craufurd, D. Neary, F. Owen, B. Oostra, J. Hardy, A. Goate, J. van Swieten, D. Mann, T. Lynch, and P. Heutink. Association of missense and 5-splice-site mutations in tau with the inherited ftdp-17. *Nature*, 393:702–705, 1998.

[51] J.S. Goldman, J.M. Farmer, E.M. Wood, J.K. Johnson, A. Boxer, J. Neuhaus, C. Lomen-Hoerth, K.C. Wilhelmsen, V.M. Lee, M. Grossman, and B.L. Miller. Comparison of family histories in ftld subtypes and related tauopathies. *Neurology*, 65:1817–1819, 2005.

[52] M. Cruts, I. Gijselinck, J. van der Zee, S. Engelborghs, H. Wils, D. Pirici, R. Rademakers, R. Vandenberghe, B. Dermaut, J.J. Martin, C. van Duijn, K. Peeters, R. Sciot, P. Santens, T. De Pooter, M. Mattheijssens, M. Van den Broeck, I. Cuijt, K. Vennekens, P.P. De Deyn, S. Kumar-Singh, and C. Van Broeckhoven. Progranulin gene mutations associated with frontotemporal dementia and progressive non-fluent aphasia. *Nature*, 442:920–924, 2006.

[53] M. Baker, I. Mackenzie, S. Pickering-Brown, J. Gass, R. Rademakers, C. Lindholm, J. Snowden, J. Adamson, A. Sadovnick, S. Rollinson, A. Cannon, E. Dwosh, D. Neary, S. Melquist, A. Richardson, D. Dickson, Z. Berger, J. Eriksen, T. Robinson, C. Zehr, C. Dickey, R. Crook, R. McGowan, D. Mann, B. Boeve, H. Feldman, and M. Hutton. Mutation in progranulin cause tau-negative frontotemporal dementia linked to chromosome 17. *Nature*, 24:916–919, 2006.

[54] J.S. Snowden, S.M. Pickering-Brown, I.R. Mackenzie, A.M. Richardson, A. Varma, D. Neary, and D.M. Mannn. Progranulin gene mutations associated with frontotemporal dementia and progressive non-fluent aphasia. *Brain*, 129:3091–3102, 2006.

[55] C.J. Mummery, K. Patterson, R. Wise, R. Vandenberghe, C.J. Price, and J. Hodges. Disrupted temporal lobe connections in semantic dementia. *Brain*, 122:61–73, 1999.

[56] J.C. Morris, M. Storandt, J.P. Miller, D.W. McKeel, J.L. Price, E.H. Rubin, and L. Berg. Mild cognitive impairment represents early-stage Alzheimer's disease. *Arch Neurol*, 58:397–405, 2001.

[57] M.A. Lambon-Ralph, K. Patterson, N. Graham, K. Dawson, and J.R. Hodges. Homogeneity and heterogeneity in mild cognitive impairment and Alzheimer's disease: a cross-sectional and longitudinal study of 55 cases. *Brain*, 126:2350–2362, 2003.

[58] R.C. Petersen, R.G. Thomas, M. Grundman, D. Bennett, R. Doody, S. Ferris, D. Galasko, S. Jin, J. Kaye, A. Levey, E. Pfeiffer, M. Sano, C.H. van Dyck, and L.J. Thal. Vitamine E and donepezil for the treatment of mild cognitive impairment. *New Engl J Med*, in press, 2005.

[59] R.C. Petersen. Mild cognitive impairment as a diagnostic entity. *J Intern Med*, 256:183–194, 2004.

[60] M. Grundman, R.C. Petersen, S.H. Ferris, R.G. Thomas, P.S. Aisen, D.A. Bennett, N.L. Foster, C.R. Jack, D.R. Galasko, R. Doody, J. Kaye, M. Sano, R. Mohs, S. Gauthier, H.T. Kim, S. Jin, A.N. Shultz, K. Schafer, R. Mulnard, C.H. van Dyck, J. Mintzer, E.Y. Zamrini, D. Cahn-Weiner, and L.J. Thal. Mild cognitive impairment can be distinguished from Alzheimer disease and normal aging for clinical trials. *Arch Neurol*, 61:59–66, 2004.

[61] B. Winblad, K. Palmer, M. Kivipelto, V. Jelic, L. Fratiglioni, L.O. Wahlund, A. Nordberg, L. Bäckman, M. Albert, O. Almkvist, H. Arai, H. BAsun, K. Blennow, M. De Leon, C. Decarli, T. Erkinjuntti, E. Giacobini, C. Graff, J. Hardy, C. Jack, A. Jorm, K. Ritchie, C. Van Duijn, P. Visser, and R.C. Petersen. Mild cognitive impairment - beyond controversies, towards a consensus: report of the International Working Group on Mild Cognitive Impairment. *J Intern Med*, 256:240–246, 2004.

[62] R.C. Petersen. *Mild cognitive impairment: Aging to Alzheimer's disease.* Oxford: Oxford University Press, 2003.

[63] C.R. Jack, R.C. Petersen, Y.C. Xu, P.C. O'Brien, G.E. Smith, R.J. Ivnik, B.F. Boeve, S.C. Waring, E.G. Tangalos, and E. Kokmen. Prediction of AD with MRI-based hippocampal volume in mild cognitive impairment. *Neurology*, 52:1397–1403, 1999.

[64] J.L. Price and J.C. Morris. Tangles and plaques in nondemented ageing and "pre-clinical" Alzheimer's disease. *Ann Neurol*, 45:358–368, 1999.

[65] J.H. Kordower, C. Yaping, G.T. Stebbins, S.T. DeKosky, E.J. Cochran, D. Bennett, and E.J. Mufson. Loss and atrophy of layer II entorhinal cortex neurons in elderly people with mild cognitive impairment. *Ann Neurol*, 49:202–213, 2001.

[66] M.M. Mesulam, P. Shaw, D. Mash, and S. Weintraub. Cholinergic nucleus basalis tauopathy emerges early in the aging-MCI-AD continuum. *Ann Neurol*, 55:815–828, 2004.

[67] T. Gomez-Isla, J.L. Price, D.W. McKeel, J.C. Morris, J.H. Growdon, and B.T. Hyman. Profound loss of layer II entorhinal cortex neurons occurs in very mild Alzheimer's disease. *J Neurosci*, 16:4491–4500, 1996.

[68] T.W. Mitchell, E.J. Mufson, J.A. Schneider, E.J. Cochran, J. Nissanov, L.Y. Han, J.L. Bienias, V. Lee, J.Q. Trojanowski, D.A. Bennett, and S.A. Arnold. Parahippocampal Tau pathology in healthy aging, mild cognitive impairment and early Alzheimer's disease. *Ann Neurol*, 51:182–189, 2002.

[69] W. Markesbery, F. Schmitt, R. Kryscio, D. Davis, C. Smith, and D. Wekstein. Neuropathological substrate of mild cognitive impairment. *Arch Neurol*, 63:38–46, 2006.

[70] A. Martin and P. Fedio. Word production and comprehension in Alzheimer's disease: The breakdown of semantic knowledge. *Brain Lang*, 19:124–141, 1983.

[71] K.A. Welsh, N. Butters, J.P. Hughes, R.C. Mohs, and A. Heyman. Detection and staging of dementia in Alzheimer's disease. *Arch Neurol*, 49:448–452, 1992.

[72] A. Monsch, M. Bondi, and D. Salmon et al. Comparisons of verbal fluency tasks in the detection of dementia of the Alzheimer type. *Arch Neurol*, 49:1253–1258, 1992.

[73] J.L. Locascio, J.H. Growdon, and S. Corkin. Cognitive test performance in detecting, staging and tracking Alzheimer's disease. *Arch Neurol*, 52:1087–1099, 1995.

[74] V.O.B. Emery. Language functioning. In R.G. Morris, editor, *The cognitive neuropsychology of Alzheimer-type dementia*, pages 166–192. Oxford University Press, Oxford, 1996.

[75] F.J. Huff, S. Corkin, and J.H. Growdon. Semantic impairment and anomia in Alzheimer's disease. *Brain Lang*, 28:235–249, 1986.

[76] H. Chertkow and D. Bub. Semantic memory loss in dementia of Alzheimer's type. *Brain*, 113:397–417, 1990.

[77] J.R. Hodges, D.P. Salmon, and N. Butters. The nature of the naming deficit in Alzheimer's and Huntington's disease. *Brain*, 114:1547–1558, 1991.

[78] H. Chertkow, D. Bub, and D. Caplan. Constraining theories of semantic memory processing: Evidence from dementia. *Cognit Neuropsychol*, 9:327–365, 1992.

[79] J.R. Hodges, D.P. Salmon, and N. Butters. Semantic memory impairment in Alzheimer's disease: Failure of access or degraded knowledge? *Neuropsychologia*, 30:301–314, 1992.

[80] J.R. Hodges and K. Patterson. Is semantic memory consistently impaired early in the course of Alzheimer's disease? neuroanatomical and diagnostic implications. *Neuropsychologia*, 33:441–459, 1995.

[81] M.A. Lambon-Ralph, K. Patterson, and J.R. Hodges. The relationship between naming and semantic knowledge for different categories in dementia of Alzheimer's type. *Neuropsychologia*, 35:1251–1260, 1997.

[82] S.A. Small, Y. Stern, M. Tang, and R. Mayeux. Selective decline in memory function among healthy elderly. *Neurology*, 52:1392–1396, 1999.

[83] M.M. Machulda, H.A. Ward, B. Borowski, J.L. Gunter, R.H. Cha, P.C. O'Brien, R.C. Petersen, B.F. Boeve, D. Knopman, D.F. Tang-Wai, R.J. Ivnik, G.E. Smith, E.G. Tangalos, and C.R. Jack. Comparison of memory fMRI response among normal, MCI and Alzheimer's patients. *Neurology*, 61:500–506, 2003.

[84] S.C. Johnson, L.C. Baxter, L. Susskind-Wilder, D.J. Connor, M.N. Sabbagh, and R.J. Caselli. Hippocampal adaptation to face repetition in healthy elderly and mild cognitive impairment. *Neuropsychologia*, 42:980–989, 2004.

[85] B.C. Dickerson, D.H. Salat, J.F. Bates, M. Atiya, R.J. Killiany, D.N. Greve, A.M. Dale, C.E. Stern, D. Blacker, M.S. Albert, and R.A. Sperling. Medial temporal function and structure in mild cognitive impairment. *Ann Neurol*, 56:27–35, 2004.

[86] B.C. Dickerson, D.H. Salat, D.N. Greve, E.F. Chua, E. Rand-Giovannetti, D. Rentz, L. Bertram, K. Mullen, R.E. Tanzi, D. Blacker, M.S. Albert, and R.A. Sperling. Increased hippocampal activation in mild cognitive impairment compared to normal aging and AD. *Neurology*, 65:404–411, 2005.

[87] M. Grossman, P. Koenig, G. Glosser, C. DeVita, P. Moore, J. Rhee, J. Detre, D. Alsop, and J. Gee. Neural basis for semantic memory difficulty in Alzheimer's disease: an fMRI study. *Brain*, 126:292–311, 2003.

[88] C.L. Grady, A.R. McIntosh, S. Beig, M.L. Keightley, H. Burian, and S.E. Black. Evidence from functional neuroimaging of a compensatory prefrontal network in Alzheimer's disease. *J Neurosci*, 23:986–993, 2003.

[89] N. Cals, G. Devuyst, G.N. Afsar, T. Karapanayiotides, and J. Bogousslavsky. Pure superficial posterior cerebral artery territory infarction in the lausanne stroke registry. *J Neurol*, 249:855–861, 2002.

[90] J. Riddoch and G. Humphreys. A case of integrative visual agnosia. *Brain*, 110:1431–1462, 1987.

[91] R.I. Rumiati and G.W. Humphreys. Visual object agnosia without alexia or prosopagnosia: Arguments for separate knowledge stores. *Visual Cognition*, 4:207–217, 1997.

[92] E. De Renzi and C. Saetti. Associative agnosia and optic aphasia: Qualitative and quantitative differences. *Cortex*, 33:115–130, 1997.

[93] L. Cohen, O. Martinaud, C. Lemer, S. Lehericy, Y. Samson, M. Obadia, A. Slachevsky, and S. Dehaene. Visual word recognition in the left and right hemispheres: anatomical and functional correlates of peripheral alexias. *Cereb Cortex*, 13:1313–1333, 2003.

[94] A. Kleinschmidt and L. Cohen. The neural bases of prosopagnosia and pure alexia: recent insights from functional neuroimaging. *Curr Opin Neurol*, 19:911–922, 2006.

[95] A.R. Damasio, H. Damasio, and G.W. Van Hoesen. Prosopagnosia: anatomical basis and behavioral mechanism. *Neurology*, 32:331–341, 1982.

[96] E. De Renzi, P. Faglioni, D. Grossi, and P. Nichelli. Apperceptive and associative forms of prosopagnosia. *Cortex*, 27:213–221, 1991.

[97] A.R. Damasio, T. Yamada, H. Damasio, J. Corbett, and J. McKee. Central achromatopsia: Behavioral, anatomic and phyiological aspects. *Neurology*, 30:1064–1071, 1980.

[98] S. Zeki. A century of cerebral achromatopsia. *Brain*, 113:1721–1777, 1991.

[99] J. Powell and J. Davidoff. Selective impairments of object knowledge in a case of acquired color blindness. *Memory*, 3:435–461, 1995.

[100] R. Gaillard, L. Naccache, P. Pinel, S. Clemenceau, E. Volle, D. Hasboun, S. Dupont, M. Baulac, S. Dehaene, C. Adam, and L. Cohen. Direct intracranial, fmri, and lesion evidence for the causal role of left inferotemporal cortex in reading. *Neuron*, 50:191–204, 2006.

[101] P. Graets, R. DeBleser, and K. Willmes. *Akense Afasie Test.* Lisse, NL: Swets and Zeitlinger, 1992.

[102] J. Kay, R. Lesser, and M. Coltheart. *Psycholinguistic assessment of language processing in aphasia.* Hove, UK: Lawrence Erlbaum Associates Ltd, 1992.

[103] R. Bastiaanse, M. Bosje, and E.G. Visch-Brink. *Psycholinguïstische testbatterij voor de taalverwerking van Afasiepatiënten (PALPA).* Hove, UK: Lawrence-Erlbaum Associates, 1995.

[104] E. Kaplan, H. Goodglass, and S. Weintraub. *The Boston Naming Test.* Lea and Febiger, Philadelphia, 1983.

[105] P. Marien, E. Mampaey, A. Vervaet, J. Saerens, and P.P. De Deyn. Normative data for the Boston Naming test in native Dutch-speaking Belgian elderly. *Brain Lang*, 65:447–467, 1998.

[106] M.J. Riddoch and G.W. Humphreys. *Birmingham Object Recognition Battery.* Hove, UK: Lawrence Erlbaum Associates Ltd, 1993.

[107] E.K. Warrington and M. James. *Visual Object and Space Perception Battery.* Thamys Valley Test Company Ltd., 1991.

[108] W. Halstead. *Brain and Intelligence.* Chicago: University of Chicago Press, 1947.

[109] J.C. Raven. *Coloured Progressive Matrices.* London: H.K. Lewis, 1962.

[110] A. Rey. *Léxamen clinique en psychologie.* Paris: Press Universitaires de France, 1964.

[111] R.J. Ivnik, J.F. Malec, E.G. Tangalos, R.C. Petersen, E. Kokmen, and L.T. Kurland. The Auditory Verbal Learning test (AVLT): Norms for ages 55 years and older. *Psychol Assess*, 2:304–312, 1990.

[112] E. Lannoo and G. Vingerhoets. Flemish normative data on common neuropsychological tests: influence of age, education and gender. *Psychologica Belgica*, 37:141–156, 1997.

[113] E. Warrington and T. Shallice. Category specific semantic impairments. *Brain*, 107:829–853, 1984.

[114] E.K. Warrington and R. McCarthy. Categories of knowledge: Further fractionations and an attempted integration. *Brain*, 110:1273–1296, 1987.

[115] E. Warrington and R. McCarthy. Multiple meaning systems in the brain: a case for visual semantics. *Neuropsychologia*, 32:1465–1473, 1994.

[116] M.J. Farah and J.L. McClelland. A computational model of semantic memory impairment: modality specificity and emergent category specificity. *J Exp Psychol Gen*, 120:339–357, 1991.

[117] A. Caramazza, A. Hillis, B. Rapp, and C. Romani. The multiple semantics hypothesis: Multiple confusions? *Cognitive Neuropsychology*, 7:161–189, 1990.

[118] S.L. Small, J. Hart, T. Nguyen, and B. Gordon. Distributed representations of semantic knowledge in the brain. *Brain*, 118:441–453, 1995.

[119] H.E. Moss, L.K. Tyler, and F. Jennings. When leopards lose ther spots: Knowledge of visual properties in category-specific deficits for living things. *Cognitive neuropsychology*, 14:901–950, 1997.

[120] A. Caramazza and J.R. Shelton. Domain specific knowledge systems in the brain: The animate-inanimate distinction. *J Cogn Neurosci*, 10:1–34, 1998.

[121] S. Cappa, D. Perani, T. Schnur, M. Tettamanti, and F. Fazio. The effects of semantic category and knowledge type on lexical-semantic access: a pet study. *Neuroimage*, 8:350–359, 1998.

[122] A. Caramazza. The organization of conceptual knowledge in the brain. In M. Gazzaniga, editor, *The new cognitive neurosciences*, pages 1037–1046. MIT Press, Cambridge, MA, 2000.

[123] L.K. Tyler and H.E. Moss. Towards a distributed account of conceptual knowledge. *Trends in Cognitive Sciences*, 5:244–252, 2001.

[124] B. Mahon and A. Caramazza. Constraining questions about the organisation and representation of conceptual knowledge. *Cognitive Neuropsychology*, 20:433–450, 2003.

[125] U. Noppeney and C. Price. Functional imaging of the semantic system: Retrieval of sensory-experienced and verbally learned knowledge. *Brain and Language*, 84:120–133, 2003.

[126] E. Warrington. The selective impairment of semantic memory. *Quart J Exp Psychol*, 27:635–657, 1975.

[127] J.S. Snowden, P.J. Goulding, and D. Neary. Semantic dementia: a form of circumscribed cerebral atrophy. *Behav Neurol*, 2:167–182, 1989.

[128] D. Howard and K. Patterson. *Pyramids and palm trees: a test of semantic access from pictures and words.* Thames Valley Publishing, 1992.

[129] J. Snodgrass and M. Vanderwart. A standardized set of 260 pictures: norms for name agreement, image agreement, familiarity and visual complexity. *J Exp Psychol Hum Learn Mem*, 6:174–215, 1980.

[130] J. te Linde. Picture-word differences in decision latency: a test of common-coding assumptions. *J Exp Psychol Learn Mem Cognit*, 8:584–598, 1982.

[131] R. Vandenberghe, P. Dupont, B. De Bruyn, G. Bormans, J. Michiels, L. Mortelmans, and G. Orban. The influence of stimulus location on the brain activation pattern in detection and orientation discrimination. *Brain*, 119:1263–1276, 1996.

[132] A. Martin and L.L. Chao. Semantic memory and the brain: structure and processes. *Curr Opin Neurobiol*, 2:194–201, 2001.

[133] A.D. Wagner, E.J. Pare-Blagoev, J. Clark, and R.A. Poldrack. Recovering meaning: Left prefrontal cortex guides controlled semantic retrieval. *Neuron*, 31:329–338, 2001.

[134] J.R. Binder, J.A. Frost, T.A. Hammeke, P.S.F. Bellgowan, S.M. Rao, and R.W. Cox. Conceptual processing during the conscious resting state: A functional MRI study. *J Cognit Neurosci*, 11:80–93, 1999.

[135] C. Lustig, A.Z. Snyder, M. Bhakta, K.C. O'Brien, M. McAvoy, M.E. Raichle, J.C. Morris, and R.L. Buckner. Functional deactivations: Change with age and dementia of the Alzheimer type. *Proc Nat Acad Sci*, 100:14504–14509, 2003.

[136] G. Sartori and R. Job. The oyster with four legs: A neuropsychological study on the interaction between vision and semantic information. *Cognitive Neuropsychology*, 5:105–132, 1988.

[137] C. Luzzatti and J. Davidoff. Impaired retrieval of object-colour knowledge with preserved colour naming. *Neuropsychologia*, 32:933–950, 1994.

[138] S.D. Breedin, E.M. Saffran, and H.B. Coslett. Reversal of the concreteness effet in a patient with semantic dementia. *Cognit Neuropsychology*, 11:617–660, 1994.

[139] S. Carbonnel, A. Charnallet, D. David, and J. Pellat. One or several semantic systems? Maybe none: Evidence from a case study of modality and category-specific "semantic" impairment. *Cortex*, 33:391–417, 1997.

[140] G. Miceli, E. Fouch, R. Capasso, J.R. Shelton, F. Tomaiuolo, and A. Caramazza. The dissociation of color from form and function knowledge. *Nature Neurosci*, 4:662–667, 2001.

[141] A.E. Hillis and A. Caramazza. Category-specific naming and comprehension impairment: A double dissociation. *Brain*, 114:2081–2094, 1991.

[142] J. Hart and B. Gordon. Neural subsystems for object knowledge. *Nature*, 359:60–64, 1992.

[143] A. Hillis. Neuroanatomical aspects of naming. In A. Hillis, editor, *The handbook of adult language disorders*, pages 143–161. Psychology Press, New York, NY, 2002.

[144] D. Chialant, A. Costa, and A. Caramazza. Neuroanatomical aspects of naming. In A. Hillis, editor, *The handbook of adult language disorders*, pages 143–161. Psychology Press, New York, NY, 2002.

[145] C.J. Price, J.T. Devlin, C.J. Moore, C. Morton, and A.R. Laird. Meta-analyses of object naming: effect of baseline. *Human Brain Mapping*, 25:70–82, 2005.

[146] C.J. Price, E. McCrory, U. Noppeney, A. Mechelli, C.J. Moore, N. Biggio, and J.T. Devlin. How reading differs from object naming at the neuronal level. *Neuroimage*, 29:643–648, 2006.

[147] A. Caramazza. How many levels of processing are there in lexical access? *Cogn Neuropsychol*, 14:177–208, 1997.

[148] C.J. Price, C.J. Moore, G.W. Humphreys, and R.J.S. Wise. Segragating semantic from phonological processing. *J Cogn Neuroscience*, 9:727–733, 1997.

[149] C.J. Fiebach, A.D. Friederici, K. Müller, and D. Yves von Cramon. fMRI evidence for dual routes to the mental lexicon in visual word recognition. *J Cognitive Neurosci*, 14:11–23, 2002.

[150] R.J.S. Wise, F. Chollet, U. Hadar, K. Friston, E. Hoffner, and R. Frackowiak. Distribution of cortical neural networks involved in word comprehension and word retrieval. *Brain*, 114:1803–1817, 1991.

[151] C.J. Price. The functional anatomy of word comprehension and production. *Trends Cogn Sci*, 2:281–288, 1998.

[152] J.R. Binder, J.A. Frost, T.A. Hammeke, P.S.F. Bellgowan, J.A. Springer, J.N. Kaufman, and E.T. Possing. Human temporal lobe activation by speech and nonspeech sounds. *Cerebral cortex*, 10:512–528, 2000.

[153] M.H. Davis, F. Meunier, and W.D. Marslen-Wilson. Neural responses to morphological, syntactic, and semantic properties of single words: An fMRI study. *Brain Lang*, 89:439–449, 2004.

[154] A.N. Herbster, M.A. Mintun, R.D. Nebes, and J.T. Becker. Regional cerebral blood flow during word and nonword reading. *Human Brain Mapping*, 5:84–92, 1997.

[155] J.A. Fiez and S.E. Petersen. Neuroimaging studies of reading. *PNAS*, 95:914–921, 1998.

[156] A. Mechelli, J. Crinion, S. Long, K. Friston, M. Lambon Ralph, K. Patterson, J. McClelland, and C. Price. Dissociating reading processes on the basis of neuronal interactions. *J Cogn Neurosci*, 17:1753–1765, 2005.

[157] J.A. Fiez, D. Tranel, D. Seager-Frerichs, and H. Damasio. Specific reading and phonological processing deficits are associated with damage to the left frontal operculum. *Cortex*, 42:624–643, 2006.

[158] G.W. Humphreys, C.J. Price, and M.J. Riddoch. From objects to names: a cognitive neuroscience approach. *Psychol Res*, 62:118–130, 1999.

[159] C. Whatmough and H. Chertkow. Neuroanatomical aspects of naming. In A. Hillis, editor, *The handbook of adult language disorders*, pages 143–161. Psychology Press, New York, NY, 2002.

[160] A. Hillis and A. Tuffiash. Neuroanatomical aspects of naming. In A. Hillis, editor, *The handbook of adult language disorders*, pages 143–161. Psychology Press, New York, NY, 2002.

[161] W. Wickelgren. Speed accuracy tradeoff and information processing dynamics. *Acta Psychol*, 41:67–85, 1977.

[162] P. Verhaeghen, A. Vandenbroucke, and V. Dierckx. Growing slower and less accurate: Adult age differences in time-accuracy functions for recall and recognition from episodic memory. *Exp Aging Res*, 24:3–19, 1998.

[163] U. Noppeney and C. Price. Retrieval of visual, auditory and abstract semantics. *NeuroImage*, 15:917–926, 2002.

[164] U. Noppeney and C. Price. Retrieval of abstract semantics. *NeuroImage*, 22:164–170, 2004.

[165] W. Glaser and F.J. Dungelhoff. The time course of picture-word interference. *J Exp Psychol Hum Percept Perform*, 10:640–654, 1984.

[166] F.X. Alario, J. Segui, and L. Ferrand. Semantic and associative priming in picture naming. *Quart J Exp Psychol*, 53A:741–764, 2000.

[167] G.S. Dell. A spreading-activation theory of retrieval in sentence production. *Psychol Rev*, 93:283–321, 1986.

[168] M. Laiacona and E. Capitani. A case of prevailing deficit of nonliving categories or a case of prevailing sparing of living categories. *Cognitive Neuropsychology*, 18:39–70, 2001.

[169] A. Villringer and U. Dirnagl. Coupling of brain activity and cerebral blood flow: basis of functional neuroimaging. *Cerebrovasc Brain Metabol Rev*, 7:240–276, 1995.

[170] A. Grinvald, T. Bonhoeffer, D. Malonek, D. Shoham, E. Bartfeld, A. Arieli, R. Hildesheim, and E. Ratzlaff. *Memory: organization and locus of change*. New York: Oxford University Press, 1991.

[171] N.K. Logothetis, J. Pauls, M. Augath, T. Trinath, and A. Oeltermann. Neurophysiological investigation of the basis of the fmri signal. *Nature*, 412:150–157, 2001.

[172] A. Hess, D. Stiller, T. Kaulisch, P. Heil, and H. Scheich. New insights into the hemodynamic blood oxygenation level-dependent response through combination of functional magnetic resonance imaging and optical recording in gerbil barrel cortex. *J Neurosci*, 20:3328–3338, 2000.

[173] J.T. Devlin, R.P. Russell, M.H. Davis, C.J. Price, J. Wilson, H.E. Moss, P.M. Matthews, and L.K. Tyler. Susceptibility-induced loss of signal: Comparing PET and fMRI on a semantic task. *NeuroImage*, 11:589–600, 2000.

[174] M. Vandenbulcke, R. Peeters, P. Van Hecke, and R. Vandenberghe. Anterior temporal laterality in primary progressive aphasia shifts to the right. *Ann Neurol*, 58:362–370, 2005.

[175] G.B. Williams, P.J. Nestor, and J.R. Hodges. Neural correlates of semantic and behavioural deficits in frontotemporal dementia. *Neuroimage*, 24:1042–1051, 2005.

[176] A.W. Song, C.A. Popp, J. Mao, and W.T. Dixon. fmri: Methodology, acquisition and processing. *Adv Neurol*, 83:177–185, 2000.

[177] M.A. Griswold, P.M. Jakob, R.M. Heidemann, M. Nittka, V. Jellus, J. Wang, B. Kiefer, and A. Haase. Generalized autocalibrating partially parallel acquisitions (GRAPPA). *Magn Reson Med*, 47:1202–1210, 2002.

[178] D.K. Sodickson and W.J. Manning. Simultaneous acquisition of spatial harmonics (smash): Fast imaging with radiofrequency coil arrays. *Magn Reson Med*, 38:591–603, 1997.

[179] R. Peeters, M. Vandenbulcke, R. Vandenberghe, and P. Van Hecke. Visualizing anterior temporal activation during semantic processing with parallel imaging techniques. *Twelfth scientific meeting and exhibition of the ISMRM*, page 739, 2004.

[180] K. Friston, A. Holmes, K. Worsley, J. Poline, C. Frith, J. Heather, and R. Frackowiak. Statistical parametric maps in functional imaging: a general approach. *Human Brain Mapping*, 2:189–210, 1995.

[181] F. Maes, A. Collignon, D. Vandermeulen, G. Marchal, and P. Suetens. Multimodality image registration by maximization of mutual information. *IEEE Transactions on Medical Imaging*, 16:187–198, 1997.

[182] J. Talairach and P. Tournoux. *Co-planar stereotaxic atlas of the human brain.* Thieme Medical Publishers, Inc, New York, 1988.

[183] F. Kherif, J.B. Poline, S. Mériaux, H. Benali, G. Flandin, and M. Brett. Group analysis in functional neuroimaging: selecting subjects using similarity measures. *NeuroImage*, 20:2197–2208, 2003.

[184] J. Ashburner and K.J. Friston. Voxel-based morphometry: The methods. *NeuroImage*, 11:805–821, 2000.

[185] C.D. Good, I.S. Johnsrude, J. Ashburner, R.N. Henson, K.J. Friston, and R.S.J. Frackowiak. A voxel-based morphometric study of ageing in 465 normal adult human brains. *Neuroimage*, 14:21–36, 2001.

[186] C.D. Good, R.I. Scahill, N.C. Fox, J. Ashburner K.J., Friston, D. Chan, W.R. Crum, M.N. Rossor, and R.S. Frackowiak RS. Automatic differentiation of anatomical patterns in the human brain: validation with studies of degenerative dementias. *Neuroimage*, 17:29–46, 2002.

[187] G. Chetelat, B. Landeau, F. Eustache, F. Mezenge, F. Viader, V. de la Sayette, B. Desgranges, and J.C. Baron. Using voxel-based morphometry to map the structural changes associated with rapid conversion in mci: A longitudinal mri study. *Neuroimage*, 27:934–946, 2005.

[188] M. Corbetta, M. Kincade, C. Lewis, A. Snyder, and A. Sapir. Neural basis and recovery of spatial attention deficits in spatial neglect. *Nat Neurosci*, 8:1603–1610, 2005.

[189] C.J. Price and K.J. Friston. Degeneracy and cognitive anatomy. *Trends Cogn Sciences*, 6:416–421, 2002.

[190] U. Noppeney, K. Friston, and C. Price. Degenerate neuronal systems sustaining cognitive functions. *J Anat*, 205:433–442, 2004.

[191] C.J. Price and J. Crinion. The latest on functional imaging of aphasic stroke. *Curr Opin Neurol*, 18:429–434, 2005.

[192] J. Crinion and C.J. Price. Right anterior superior temporal activation predicts auditory sentence comprehension following aphasic stroke. *Brain*, 128:2858–2871, 2005.

[193] C. Price and K. Friston. Scanning patients with tasks they can perform. *Hum Brain Mapp*, 8:102–108, 1999.

[194] E. Salmon. Functional brain imaging applications to the differential diagnosis in the dementias. *Curr Opin Neurol*, 15:439–444, 2002.

[195] D.S. Knopman, A.B. Rubens, O.A. Selnes, A.C. Klassen, and M.W. Meyer. Mechanisms of recovery from aphasia: Evidence from serial Xenon 133 cerebral blood flow studies. *Ann Neurol*, 15:530–535, 1984.

[196] C. Weiller, C. Isensee, M. Rijntjes, W. Huber, S. Muller, D. Bier, K. Dutschka, R.P. Woods, J. Noth, and H.C. Diener. Recovery from Wernicke's aphasia: a positron emission tomography study. *Ann Neurol*, 37:723–732, 1995.

[197] P. Belin, P. Van Eeckhout, M. Zilbovicius, P. Remy, C. Francois, S. Guillaume, F. Chain, G. Rancurel, and Y. Samson. Recovery from nonfluent aphasia after melodic intonation therapy: a PET study. *Neurology*, 47:1504–1511, 1996.

[198] K.R. Thulborn, P.A. Carpenter, and M.A. Just. Plasticity of language-related brain function during recovery from stroke. *Stroke*, 30:749–754, 1999.

[199] Y. Cao, E.M. Vikingstad, K.P. George, A.F. Johnson, and K.M.A. Welch. Cortical language activation in stroke patients recovering from aphasia with functional MRI. *Stroke*, 30:2331–2340, 1999.

[200] H.J. Rosen, S.E. Petersen, M.R. Linenweber, A.Z. Snyder, D.A. White, L. Chapman, A.W. Dromerick, J.A. Fiez, and M. Corbetta. Neural correlates of recovery from aphasia after damage to left inferior frontal cortex. *Neurology*, 55:1883–1894, 2000.

[201] A.E. Hillis. Does the right make it right? *Ann Neurol*, 51:537–538, 2002.

[202] A. Leff, J. Crinion, S. Scott, F. Turkheimer, D. Howard, and R. Wise. A physiological change in the homotopic cortex following left posterior temporal lobe infarction. *Ann Neurol*, 51:553–558, 2002.

[203] L. Bartha, E. Trinka, M. Ortler, E. Donnemiller, S. Felber, G. Bauer, and T. Benke. Linguistic deficits following left selective amygdalohippocampectomy: a prospective study. *Epilepsy Behav*, 5:348–357, 2004.

[204] V. Blasi, A.C. Young, A.P. Tansy, S.E. Petersen, and A.Z. Snyder. Word retrieval learning modulates right frontal cortex in patients with left frontal damage. *Neuron*, 36:159–170, 2002.

[205] A.E. Hillis. Can shift to the right be a good thing? *Ann Neurol*, 58:346–347, 2005.

[206] O.A. Selnes. The corpus callosum: Some anatomical and functional considerations with special reference to language. *Brain Lang*, 1:111–139, 1974.

[207] H. Karbe, A. Thiel, G. Weber-Luxenburger, K. Herholz, J. Kessler, and W.D. Heiss. Brain plasticity in poststroke aphasia: What is the contribution of the right hemisphere? *Brain Language*, 64:215–230, 1998.

[208] W.D. Heiss, J. Kessler, A. Thiel, M. Ghaemi, and H. Karbe. Differential capacity of left and right hemispheric areas for compensation of poststroke aphasia. *Ann Neurol*, 45:430–438, 1999.

[209] E. Zaidel. Auditory vocabulary of the right hemisphere following brain bisection or hemidecortication. *Cortex*, 12:191–211, 1976.

[210] G. Gainotti. The riddle of the right hemisphere's contribution to the recovery of language. *Eur J Disord Communic*, 28:227–246, 1993.

[211] C.A. Marczinski, W. Davidson, and A. Kertesz. A longitudinal study of behavior in frontotemporal dementia and primary progressive aphasia. *Cogn Behav Neurol*, 17:185–190, 2004.

[212] A. Thiel, B. Habedank, L. Winhuisen, K. Herholz, J. Kessler, W.F. Haupt, and W.D. Heiss. Essential language function of the right hemisphere in brain tumor patients. *Ann Neurol*, 57:128–131, 2005.

[213] M. Cotelli, R. Manenti, S. Cappa, C. Geroldi, O. Zanetti, P. Rossini, and C. Miniussi. Effect of transcranial magnetis stimulation on action naming in patients with alzheimer disease. *Arch Neurol*, 63:1602–1604, 2006.

[214] M. Musso, C. Weiller, S. Kiebel, S.P. Müller, P. Bülau, and M. Rijntjens. Training-induced brain plasticity in aphasia. *Brain*, 122:1781–1790, 1999.

[215] E. Seto, G. Sela, W.E. McIlroy, S.E. Black, and W.R. Staines. Quantifying head motion associated with motor tasks used in fmri. *Neuroimage*, 14:284–297, 2001.

[216] K.J. Friston, A. Holmes, J.B. Poline, J. Grasby, S.C. Williams, R.S. Frackowiak, and R. Turner. Analysis of fmri time-series revisited. *Neuroimage*, 2:45–53, 1995.

[217] K.J. Friston, S.C. Williams, R. Howard, R.S. Frackowiak, and R. Turner. Movement-related effects in fmri time-series. *Magn Reson Med*, 35:346–355, 1996.

[218] M. Brett, A.P. Leff, C. Rorden, and J. Ashburner. Spatial normalization of brain images with focal lesions using cost function masking. *Neuroimage*, 14:486–500, 2001.

[219] M. Vandenbroucke, R. Goekoop, E. Duschek, J. Netelenbos, J. Kuijer, F. Barkhof, P. Scheltens, and S. Rombouts. Interindividual differences of medial temporal lobe activation during encoding in an elderly population studied by fmri. *NeuroImage*, 21:173–180, 2004.

[220] S. Krishnan, M.J. Slavin, T.T. Tran, P.M. Doraiswamy, and J.R. Petrella. Accuracy of spatial normalization of the hippocampus: Implications for fmri research in memory disorders. *NeuroImage*, 31:560–571, 2006.

[221] K. Baete, J. Nuyts, W. Van Paesschen, S. Ceyssens, L. De Ceuninck, O. Gheysens, A. Kelles, J. Van den Eynden, P. Suetens, and P. Dupont. Evaluation of anatomy based reconstruction for partial volume correction in brain fdg-pet. *NeuroImage*, 23:305–317, 2004.

[222] M. D'Esposito, L.Y. Deouell, and A. Gazzaley. Alterations in the BOLD fMRI signal with ageing and disease: A challenge for neuroimaging. *Nature Rev Neurosci*, 4:863–872, 2003.

[223] S.C. Blank, H. Bird, F. Turkheimer, and R.J.S. Wise. Speech production after stroke: The role of the right pars opercularis. *Ann Neurol*, 54:310–320, 2003.

[224] A. Thiel, K. Herholz, A. Koyuncu, M. Ghaemi, L.W. Kracht, B. Habedank, and W.D. Heiss. Plasticity of language networks in patients with brain tumors: a positron emission tomography study. *Ann Neurol*, 50:620–629, 2001.

[225] R.C. Oldfield. The assessment and analysis of handedness: The Edinburgh inventory. *Neuropsychologia*, 9:87–113, 1971.

[226] R.C. Petersen, J.C. Stevens, M. Ganguli, E.G. Tangalos, J.L. Cummings, and S.T. DeKosky. Practice parameter: mild cognitive impairment (an evidence-based review). *Neurology*, 56:1133–1142, 2001.

[227] S.C. Cramer, G. Nelles, R.R. Benson, J.D. Kaplan, R.A. Parker, K.K. Kwong, D.N. Kennedy, S.P. Finklestein, and B.R. Rosen. A functional MRI study of subjects recovered from hemiparetic stroke. *Stroke*, 28:2518–2527, 1997.

[228] A. Basso, M. Gardelli, M.P. Grassi, and M. Mariotti. The role of the right hemisphere in recovery from aphasia. two case studies. *Cortex*, 25:555–566, 1989.

[229] A. Kertesz. *Aphasia and associated disorders*. Grune and Stratton, New York, 1979.

[230] O.A. Selnes, D.S. Knopman, N. Niccum, A.B. Rubens, and D. Larson. Computed tomographic scan correlates of auditory comprehension deficits in aphasia: a prospecitive recovery study. *Ann Neurol*, 13:558–566, 1983.

[231] D.S. Knopman, O.L. Selnes, N. Niccum, A.B. Rubens, D. Yock, and D. Larson. A longitudinal study of speech fluency in aphasia: CT correlates of recovery and persistent nonfluency. *Neurology*, 33:1170–1178, 1983.

[232] M.S. Gazzaniga and R.W. Sperry. Language after section of the cerebral commissures. *Brain*, 90:131–138, 1967.

[233] M. Kinsbourne. The minor cerebral hemisphere as a source of aphasic speech. *Arch Neurol*, 25:302–306, 1971.

[234] J.T. Becker, M.A. Mintun, K. Aleva, M.B. Wiseman, T. Nichols, and S.T. DeKosky. Compensatory reallocation of brain resources supporting verbal episodic memory in Alzheimer's disease. *Neurology*, 46:692–700, 1996.

[235] M.F. Schwartz, O.S.M. Marin, and E.M. Saffran. Dissociations of language function in dementia: A case study. *Brain Lang*, 7:277–306, 1979.

[236] M. Grossman. Progressive aphasic syndromes: Clinical and theoretical advances. *Curr Opin Neurol*, 15:409–413, 2002.

[237] C. McMillan, J. Gee, P. Moore, K. Dennis, C. DeVita, and M. Grossman. Confrontation naming and morphometric analyses of structural MRI in frontotemporal dementia. *Dement Geriatr Cogn Disord*, 17:320–323, 2004.

[238] P.J. Nestor, N.L. Graham, T.D. Fryer, G.B. Williams, K. Patterson, and J.R. Hodges. Progressive non-fluent aphasia is associated with hypometabolism centred on the left anterior insula. *Brain*, 126:2406–2418, 2003.

[239] J.L. McClelland and T.T. Rogers. The parallel distributed processing approach to semantic cognition. *Nat Rev Neurosci*, 4:310–322, 2003.

[240] P.C. Fletcher, F. Happe, U. Frith, S.C. Baker, R.J. Dolan, R.S.J. Frackowiak, and C.D. Frith. Other minds in the brain: a functional imaging study of "theory of mind" in story comprehension. *Cognition*, 57:109–128, 1995.

[241] R. Vandenberghe, A.C. Nobre, and C.J. Price. The response of left temporal cortex to sentences. *J Cognitive Neurosci*, 14:550–560, 2002.

[242] M.M. Mesulam. From sensation to cognition. *Brain*, 121:1013–1052, 1998.

[243] G. McKhann, D. Drachman, M. Folstein, R. Katzman, D. Price, and E.M. Stadlan. Clinical diagnosis of Alzheimer's disease: report of the NINCDS-ADRDA Work group under the auspices of Department of Health and Human Services Task Force on Alzheimer's disease. *Neurology*, 34:939–994, 1984.

[244] A. Kertesz and J.B. Orange. Primary progressive aphasia: The future of neurolinguistic and biologic characterisation. *Brain Lang*, 71:116–119, 2000.

[245] D.E. Meyer and R.X. Schvaneveldt. Facilitation in recognizing pairs of words: evidence of a dependence between retrieval operations. *J Exp Psychol*, 90:227–234, 1971.

[246] W. Glaser. Picture naming. *Cognition*, 42:61–105, 1992.

[247] W. Levelt. Producing spoken language: A blueprint of the speaker. In C. Brown and P. Hagoort, editors, *The neurocognition of language*, pages 84–122. Oxford University Press, Oxford, UK, 1999.

[248] A.M. Collins and E.F. Loftus. A spreading-activation theory of semantic processing. *Psychol Rev*, 82:407–428, 1975.

[249] A. Roelofs. A spreading-activation theory of lemma retrieval in speaking. *Cognition*, 42:107–142, 1992.

[250] S.M. Park, J.D.E. Gabrieli, S. Reminger, L.A. Monti, D.A. Fleischman, R.S. Wilson, J.R. Tinklenberg, and J.A. Yesavage. Preserved priming across study-test picture transformations in patients with Alzheimer's Disease. *Neuropsychology*, 12:340–352, 1998.

[251] B. Giffard, B. Desgranges, F. Nore-Mary, C. Lalevée, V. de la Sayette, F. Pasquier, and F. Eustache. The nature of semantic memory deficits in Alzheimer's disease. New insights from hyperpriming effects. *Brain*, 124:1522–1532, 2001.

[252] H. Chertkow and D. Bub. Priming and semantic memory loss in Alzheimer's disease. *Brain Lang*, 36:420–446, 1989.

[253] B. Giffard, B. Desgranges, F. Nore-Mary, C. Lalevée, H. Beaunnieux, V. de la Sayette, F. Pasquier, and F. Eustache. The dynamic time course of semantic memory impairment in Alzheimer's disease: clues from hyperpriming and hypopriming effects. *Brain*, 125:2044–2057, 2002.

[254] S. Auchterlonie, N.A. Phillips, and H. Chertkow. Behavioral and electrical brain measures of semantic priming in patients with Alzheimer's disease: Implications for access failure versus deterioration hypothesis. *Brain Cognition*, 48:264–267, 2002.

[255] P. Marangoloa, E. DiPace, R. Rafal, and D. Scabini. Effects of parietal lesions in humans on color and location priming. *J Cognitive Neurosci*, 10:704–716, 1998.

[256] J.C. Morris, C. Ernesto, K. Schafer, M. Coats, S. Leon, M. Sano, L.J. Thal, and P. Woodbury. Clinical dementia rating training and reliability in multicenter studies: the Alzheimer's Disease Cooperative Study experience. *Neurology*, 48:1508–1510, 1997.

[257] M.F. Folstein, S.E. Folstein, and P.R. McHugh. Mini-mental state: A practical method for grading the cognitive state of patients for the clinician. *J Psychiatr Res*, 12:189–198, 1975.

[258] Kucera and W.N. Francis. *Computational analysis of present-day American English.* Brown University Press, Province, 1967.

[259] H.R. Baayen, R. Piepenbrock, and H. Van Rijn. *The CELEX lexical database (CD-ROM).* Philadelphia, PA: Linguistic Data Consortium, 1993.

[260] L.K. Tyler, H.E. Moss, K. Patterson, and J. Hodges. The gradual deterioration of syntax and semantics in a patient with progressive aphasia. *Brain Lang*, 56:426–476, 1997.

[261] J.H. Neely. Semantic priming and retrieval from lexical memory: roles of inhibitionless spreading activation and limited-capacity attention. *J Exp Psychol Gen*, 106:226–254, 1977.

[262] S.M. Rosso, L.D. Kaat, T. Baks, M. Joosse, I. de Koning, Y. Pijnenburg, D. de Jong, D. Dooijes, W. Kamphorst, R. Ravid, M.F. Niermeijer, F. Verheij, H.P. Kremer, P. Scheltens, C.M. Van Duijn, P. Heutink, and J.C. van Swieten. Frontotemporal dementia in the Netherlands: patient characteristics and prevalence estimates from a population-based study. *Brain*, 126:2016–2022, 2003.

[263] T. Blaxton and S. Bookheimer. Retrieval inhibition in anomia. *Brain Lang*, 44:221–237, 1993.

[264] J. Duncan and G.W. Humphreys. Visual search and stimulus similarity. *Psychol Rev*, 96:433–458, 1989.

[265] C. Bundesen. A theory of visual attention. *Psychol Rev*, 97:523–547, 1990.

[266] A.E. Hillis, B.C. Rapp, and A. Caramazza. When a rose is a rose in speech but a tulip in writing. *Cortex*, 35:337–356, 1999.

[267] A.E. Hillis, S. Oh, and L. Ken. Deterioration of naming nouns versus verbs in primary progressive aphasia. *Ann Neurol*, 55:268–275, 2004.

[268] M. Schwarz, R. De Bleser, K. Poeck, and J. Weis. A case of primary progressive aphasia: A 14-year follow-up study with neuropathological findings. *Brain*, 121:115–126, 1998.

[269] C. Papagno and E. Capitani. Slowly progressive aphasia: A four-year follow-up study. *Neuropsychologia*, 39:678–686, 2001.

[270] A.E. Hillis, E. Tuffiash, and A. Caramazza. Modality-specific deterioration in naming verbs in nonfluent primary progressive aphasia. *J Cognitive Neurosci*, 14:1099–1108, 2002.

[271] S. Weintraub, N.P. Rubin, and M.M. Mesulam. Primary progressive aphasia: Longitudinal course, neuropsychological profile and language features. *Arch Neurol*, 47:1329–1335, 1990.

[272] E. Le Rhun, F. Richard, and F. Pasquier. Natural history of primary progressive aphasia. *Neurology*, 65:887–891, 2005.

[273] G. Chetelat, B. Desgranges, V. de la Sayette, F. Viader, F. Eustache, and J.C. Baron. Mapping gray matter loss with voxel-based morphometry in mild cognitive impairment. *Neuroreport*, 13:1939–1943, 2002.

[274] D. Mungas, D. Harvey, B.R. Reed, W.J. Jagust, C. DeCarli, L. Beckett, W.J. Mack, J.H. Kramer, M.W. Weiner, N. Schuff, and H.C. Chui. Longitudinal volumetric mri change and rate of cognitive decline. *Neurology*, 23:565–571, 2005.

[275] C.R. Jack, R.C. Petersen, Y. Xu, P.C. O'Brien, G.E. Smith, R.J. Ivnik, B.F. Boeve, E.G. Tangalos, and E. Kokmen. Rates of hippocampal atrophy in normal aging, mild cognitive impairment and Alzheimer's disease. *Neurology*, 55:484–489, 2000.

[276] L. deToledo Morrell, T.R. Stoub, M. Bulgakova, R.S. Wilson, D.A. Bennett, S. Leurgans, J. Wuu, and D.A. Turner. Mri-derived entorhinal volume is a good predictor of conversion from mci to ad. *Neurobiol Aging*, 25:1197–1203, 2004.

[277] E.S.C. Korf, L.O. Wahlund, P.J. Visser, and P. Scheltens. Medial temporal lobe atrophy on MRI predicts dementia in patients with mild cognitive impairment. *Neurology*, 63:94–100, 2004.

[278] R.J. Killiany, T. Gomez-Isla, M. Moss, R. Kikinis, T. Sandor, F. Jolesz, R. Tanzi, K. Jones, B.T. Hyman, and M.S. Albert. Use of structural magnetic resonance imaging to predict who will get alzheimer's disease. *Ann Neurol*, 47:430–439, 2000.

[279] N.C. Fox, E.K. Warrington, P.A. Freeborough, P. Hartikainen, A.M. Kennedy, J.M. Stevens, and M.N. Rossor. Presymptomatic hippocampal atrophy in alzheimer's disease, a longitudinal mri study. *Brain*, 119:2001–2007, 1996.

[280] N.C. Fox, W.R. Crum, R.I. Scahill, J.M. Stevens, J.C. Janssen, and M.N. Rossor. Imaging of onset and progression of alzheimer's disease with voxel compression mapping of serial magnetic resonance images. *Lancet*, 358:201–205, 2001.

[281] P.M. Thompson, K.M. Hayashi, G. de Zubicaray, A.L. Janke, S.E. Rose, J. Semple, D. Herman, M.S. Hong, S.S. Dittmer, D.M. Doddrell, and A.W. Toga. Dynamics of gray matter loss in alzheimer's disease. *J Neurosci*, 23:994–1005, 2003.

[282] N.C. Fox and J.M. Schott. Imaging cerebral atrophy: Normal ageing to alzheimer's disease. *Lancet*, 363:392–394, 2004.

[283] G.B. Karas, P. Scheltens, S.A. Rombouts, P.J. Visser, R.A. van Schijndel, N.C. Fox, and F. Barkhof. Global and local gray matter loss in mild cognitive impairment and alzheimer's disease. *NeuroImage*, 23:708–716, 2004.

[284] J.M. Schott, S.L. Price, C. Frost, J.L. Whitwell, M.N. Rossor, and N.C. Fox. Measuring atrophy in alzheimer disease. a serial mri study over 6 and 12 months. *Neurology*, 65:119–124, 2005.

[285] M. Vandenbulcke, R. Peeters, P. Dupont, P. Van Hecke, and R. Vandenberghe. Word reading and posterior temporal dysfunction in amnestic mild cognitive impairment. *Cerebral cortex*, In press, 2007.

[286] M. Vandenbulcke, R. Peeters, K. Fannes, and R. Vandenberghe. Knowledge of visual attributes in the right hemisphere. *Nat Neurosci*, 9:964–970, 2006.

[287] D. Chan, N.C. Fox, R.I. Scahill, W.R. Crum, J.L. Whitwell, G. Leschziner, A.M. Rossor, J.M. Stevens, L. Cipolotti, and M.N. Rossor. Patterns of temporal lobe atrophy in semantic dementia and Alzheimer's disease. *Ann Neurol*, 49:433–442, 2001.

[288] R.R. Davies, J.R. Hodges, J.J. Kril, K. Patterson, G.M. Halliday, and J.H. Xuereb. The pathological basis of semantic dementia. *Brain*, 128:1984–1995, 2005.

[289] K. Usui, A. Ikeda, M. Takayama, M. Matsuhashi, J. Yamamoto, T. Satoh, T. Begum, N. Mikuni, J.B. Takahashi, S. Miyamoto, N. Hashimoto, and H. Shibasaki. Conversion of semantic information into phonological representation: a function in left posterior basal temporal area. *Brain*, 126:632–641, 2003.

[290] A.E. Hillis, J.T. Kleinman, M. Newhart, J. Heidler-Gary, R. Gottesman, P.B. Barker, E. Aldrich, R. Llinas, R. Wityk, and P. Chaudhry. Restoring cerebral blood flow reveals neural regions critical for naming. *J Neurosci*, 26:8069–8073, 2006.

[291] A. Martin, C. Wiggs, L. Ungerleider, and J. Haxby. Neural correlates of category-specific knowledge. *Nature*, 379:649–652, 1996.

[292] C. Price, C. Moore, and R.S.J. Frackowiak. The effect of varying stimulus rate and duration on brain activity during reading. *Neuroimage*, 3:40–52, 1996.

[293] D. Tranel, T.J. Grabowski, J. Lyon, and H. Damasio. Naming the same entities from visual or from auditory stimulation engages similar regions of left inferotemporal cortices. *J Cogn Neurosci*, 17:1239–1305, 2005.

[294] I. Ferrer. Neurons and their dendrites in frontotemporal dementia. *Dement Geriatr Cogn Disord*, 10:S35–40, 1999.

[295] M. Posner and T. Carr. Lexical access and the brain: Anatomical constraints on cognitive models of word recognition. *Am J Psychology*, 105:1–26, 1992.

[296] R. Petersen, M. Grundman, R. Thomas, and L. Thal. Donepezil and vitamin E as treatments for mild cognitive impairment. *Neurobiol Aging*, 25:S2 01–05–05, 2004.

[297] F. Cuetos, T. Martinez, C. Martinez, C. Izura, and A. Ellis. Lexical processing in spanish patients with probable alzheimer's disease. *Cogn Brain Res*, 17:549–561, 2003.

[298] K. Bayles, C. Tomoeda, A. Kaszniak, and M. Trosset. Alzheimer's disease effects on semantic memory: Loss of structure or impaired processing. *J Cogn Neurosci*, 3:166–182, 1990.

[299] R.D. Nebes and C.B. Brady. Integrity of semantic features in Alzheimer's disease. *Cortex*, 24:291–299, 1988.

[300] R.D. Nebes and C.B. Brady. Preserved organisation of semantic attributes in Alzheimer's disease. *Psychol Aging*, 5:574–579, 1990.

[301] A. Ellis and A. Young. *Human cognitive neuropsychology*. Lawrence Erlbaum, Hove, UK, 1988.

[302] American Psychiatric Association. *Diagnostic and statistical manual of mental disorders 4th ed.* American Psychiatric Association, Washington, DC, 1994.

[303] R.I. Pfeffer, T.T. Kurosaki, C.H. Harrah, J.M. Chance, and S. Filos. Measurement of functional activities in older adults in the community. *J Gerontol*, 37:323–329, 1992.

[304] T. Nichols, M. Brett, J. Andersson, T. Wager, and J.B. Poline. Valid conjunction inference with the minimum statistic. *Neuroimage*, 25:653–660, 2005.

[305] S. Larrieu, L. Letenneur, J.M. Orgogozo, C. Fabrigoule, H. Amieva, N. Le Carret, P. Barberger-Gateau, and J.F. Dartigues. Incidence and outcome of mild cognitive impairment in a population-based prospective cohort. *Neurology*, 59:1594–1599, 2002.

[306] A. Bozoki, B. Giordani, J.L. Heidebrink, S. Berent, and N.L. Foster. Mild cognitive impairments predict dementia in nondemented elderly patients with memory loss. *Arch Neurol*, 58:411–416, 2001.

[307] F. Massoud, H. Chertkow, V. Whitehead, O. Overbury, and H. Bergman. Word-reading thresholds in Alzheimer's disease and mild memory loss: A pilot study. *Alzheimer Disease and Associated Disorders*, 16:31–39, 2002.

[308] P. Tiraboschi, L.A. Hansen, L.J. Thal, and J. Corey-Bloom. The importance of neuritic plaques and tangles to the development and evolution of AD. *Neurology*, 62:1984–1989, 2004.

[309] S.Y. Bookheimer, T.A. Zeffiro, T. Blaxton, W. Gaillard, and W. Theodore. Regional cerebral blood flow during object naming and word reading. *Human Brain Mapping*, 3:93–106, 1995.

[310] L. Cohen, S. Dehaene, L. Naccache, S. Lehericy, G. Dehaene-Lambertz, M. Henaff, and F. Michel. The visual word form area: Spatial and temporal characterization of an initial stage of reading in normal subjects and posterior split brain patients. *Brain*, 123:291–307, 2000.

[311] K. McDermott, S. Petersen, J. Watson, and J. Ojemann. A procedure for identifying regions preferentially activated by attention to semantic and phonological relations using functional magnetic resonance imaging. *Neuropsychologia*, 41:293–303, 2003.

[312] S.A. Kotz, S.F. Cappa, D.Y. von Cramon, and A.D. Friederici. Modulation of the lexical-semantic network by auditory semantic priming: An event-related functional MRI study. *Neuroimage*, 17:1761–1772, 2002.

[313] J. Rissman, J.C. Eliassen, and S. E. Blumstein. An event-related fMRI investigation of implicit semantic priming. *J Cognitive Neurosci*, 15:1160–1175, 2003.

[314] B. Butterworth, D. Howard, and P. McLoughlin. The semantic deficit in aphasia: the relationship between semantic errors in auditory comprehension and picture naming. *Neuropsychologia*, 22:409–426, 1984.

[315] G. Gainotti. The status of semantic-lexical structures in anomia. *Aphasiology*, 1:449–461, 1987.

[316] J. Hart and B. Gordon. Delineation of single-word semantic comprehension deficits in aphasia, with anatomical correlation. *Ann Neurol*, 27:226–231, 1990.

[317] H. Chertkow, D. Bub, C. Deaudon, and V. Whitehead. On the status of object concepts in aphasia. *Brain Lang*, 58:203–232, 1997.

[318] M.M. Mesulam. Attentional networks, confusional states and neglect syndromes. In M.M. Mesulam, editor, *Principles of behavioral and cognitive neurology*, pages 174–256. Oxford University Press, New York, NY, 2000.

[319] A.E. Hillis, R.J. Wityk, E. Tuffiash, N.J. Beauchamp, M.A. Jacobs, P.B. Barker, and O.A. Selnes. Hypoperfusion of Wernicke's area predicts severity of semantic deficit in acute stroke. *Ann Neurol*, 50:561–566, 2001.

[320] W. Levelt and P. Indefrey. The speaking mind/brain. In A. Marantz, Y. Miyashita, and W. O'Neil, editors, *Image, language, brain*, pages 77–93. The MIT Press, London, UK, 2000.

[321] C.J. Price and A. Mechelli. Reading and reading disturbance. *Neuroimage*, 15:231–238, 2005.

[322] K.A. Bayles and C.K. Tomoeda. Confrontation naming impairment in dementia. *Brain Lang*, 19:98–114, 1983.

[323] R.D. Nebes. Semantic memory in Alzheimer's disease. *Psychol Bull*, 106:377–394, 1989.

[324] Plato. Phaedo. *http://classics.mit.edu/Plato/Phaedo.html (1994)*, 360.

[325] M. Farah. The neurological basis of mental imagery: A componential analyis. *Cognition*, 18:245–272, 1984.

[326] J. Sergent. The neuropsychology of visual image generation: Data, method, and theory. *Brain Cogn*, 13:98–129, 1990.

[327] S.M. Kosslyn and J.R. Pomerantz. Image, propositions, and the form of internal representations. *Cogn Psychol*, 9:52–76, 1977.

[328] A. Ishai, L.G. Ungerleider, and J.V. Haxby. Distributed neural systems for the generation of visual images. *Neuron*, 28:979–990, 2000.

[329] T. Shallice. *From neuropsychology to mental structure*. Cambridge: Cambridge University Press, 1988.

[330] D. Marr. *Vision*. Freeman, San Francisco, 1983.

[331] D.A. Allport. Distributed memory, modular subsystems and dysphasia. In S.K. Newman and R. Epstein, editors, *Current perspectives in dysphasia*, pages 32–60. Churchill Livingstone, Edinburgh, 1985.

[332] R. Lauro-Grotto, C. Piccini, and T. Shallice. Modality-specific operations in semantic dementia. *Cortex*, 33:593–622, 1997.

[333] J. Riddoch and G. Humphreys. Visual object processing in optic aphasia: a case of semantic access agnosia. *Cognitive Neuropsychology*, 4:131–185, 1987.

[334] N. Hadjikani and B. de Gelder. Neural basis of prosopagnosia: An fmri study. *Hum Brain Mapp*, 16:176–182, 2002.

[335] N. Hadjikani, A.K. Liu, A.M. Dale, P. Cavanagh, and R.B.H. Tootell. Retinotopy and color sensitivity in human visual cortical area v8. *Nat Neurosci*, 1:235–241, 1998.

[336] W. Ruts, S. De Deyne, E. Ameel, W. Vanpaemel, T. Verbeemen, and G. Storms. Dutch norm data for 13 semantic categories and 338 exemplars. *Behav Res Methods Instrum Comput*, 36:506–515, 2004.

[337] J.R. Crawford and D.C. Howell. Comparing an individual's test score against norms derived from small samples. *Clin Neuropsychol*, 12:482–486, 1998.

[338] J.R. Crawford and P.H. Garthwaite. Testing for suspected impairments and dissociations in single-case studies in neuropsychology: Evaluation of alternatives using monte carlo simulations and revised tests for dissociations. *Neuropsychology*, 19:318–331, 2005.

[339] P. Faglioni and C. Botti. How to differentiate retrieval from storage deficit: A stochastic approach to semantic memory modeling. *Cortex*, 29:501–518, 1993.

[340] K. Denys, W. Vanduffel, D. Fize, K. Nelissen, H. Peuskens, D. Van Essen, and G.A. Orban. The processing of visual shape in the cerebral cortex of human and nonhuman primates: a functional magnetic resonance imaging study. *J Neurosci*, 24:2551–2565, 2004.

[341] M. Farah. *Visual Agnosia*. The MIT Press, Cambridge, Massachusetts, 2004.

[342] L.L. Chao, J.V. Haxby, and A. Martin. Attribute-based neural substrates in temporal cortex for perceiving and knowing about objects. *Nat Neurosci*, 2:913–919, 1999.

[343] L.W. Barsalou. Perceptual symbol systems. *Behav Brain Sci*, 22:577–609, 1999.

[344] Z. Pylyshyn. *Seeing and visualizing: It is not what you think*. Cambridge, MA: MIT Press, 2003.

[345] R. Jackendoff. On beyond zebra: The relation of linguistic and visual information. *Cognition*, 26:89–114, 1987.

[346] A. Paivio. Dual coding theory: Retrospect and current status. *Can J Psychol*, 45:255–287, 1991.

[347] P. McKenna and E.K. Warrington. The neuropsychology of semantic memory. In F. Boller and J. Grafman, editors, *Handbook of neuropsychology*, volume 2, pages ch. 15 355–382. Elsevier Science, Amsterdam, 2000.

[348] R. McCarthy and E. Warrington. Evidence for modality-specific meaning systems in the brain. *Nature*, 334:428–430, 1988.

[349] M. Vandenbulcke, R. Peeters, K. Porke, P. Van Hecke, and R. Vandenberghe. Progression of language impairment in primary progressive aphasia: Cognitive and structural mri predictors. *Alzheimer and Dementia*, 2, 2006.

[350] R. Vandenberghe, M. Vandenbulcke, S. Weintraub, N. Johnson, K. Porke, C. Thompson, and M.M. Mesulam. Paradoxical features of word finding difficulty in primary progressive aphasia. *Ann Neurol*, 57:204–209, 2005.

[351] A.C. Nobre and G. McCarthy. Language-related field potentials in the anterior-medial temporal lobe: II. effects of word type and semantic priming. *J Neurosci*, 15:1090–1098, 1995.

[352] K. Friston, C. Buechel, G. Fink, J. Morris, E. Rolls, and R. Dolan. Psychophysiological and modulatory interaction in neuroimaging. *Neuroimage*, 6:218–229, 1997.

[353] K. Friston, L. Harrison, and W. Penny. Dynamic causal modelling. *Neuroimage*, 19:1273–1302, 2003.

[354] R. Vandenberghe, M. Vandenbulcke, P. Dupont, G. Bormans, A. Verbruggen, L. Mortelmans, and K. Van Laere. Voxel-based parametric mapping of cholinesterase activity using [11c]-pmp in mild cognitive impairment (mci). *Ann Neurol*, 56:S50, 2004.

[355] N. Nelissen, M. Vandenbulcke, P. Dupont, R. Peeters, K. Van Laere, G. Bormans, and R. Vandenberghe. Amyloid deposition and fmri activity during lexical-semantic retrieval in early stage alzheimer's disease. *Soc Neurosci Abs*, page 707.8, 2006.

[356] J. Theuns, E. Marjaux, M. Vandenbulcke, K. Van Laere, S. Kumar-Singh, G. Bormans, M. Van den Broeck, K. Vennekens, E. Corsmit, B. De Strooper, C. Van Broeckhoven, and R. Vandenberghe. Alzheimer dementia caused by a novel mutation located furthest c-terminal in app. *Human mutation*, 27:888–896, 2006.

[357] W.E. Klunk, H. Engler, A. Nordberg, Y. Wang, G. Blomqvist, D.P. Holt, M. Bergström, I. Savitcheva, G.F. Huang, S. Estrada, B. Ausen, M.L. Debnath, J. Barletta, J.C. Price, J. Sandell, B.J. Lopresti, A. Wall, P. Koivisto, G. Antoni, C.A. Mathis, and B. Langström. Imaging brain amyloid in Alzheimer's disease with Pittsburgh compound-B. *Ann Neurol*, 55:306–319, 2004.

Curriculum Vitae

Personal data

Born September 04, 1972. Belgian citizen. Married to Martine Aelbrecht June 19, 1999. Two children, Sophie, born November 10, 2000 and Victor, born December 10, 2001.

Education

- October 2002 - September 2006: Doctorate training for the degree of doctor of medical sciences, Faculty of Medicine, Katholieke Universiteit Leuven
- June 2004: Degree of Medical Doctor, Specialist in Psychiatry, Faculty of Medicine, Katholieke Universiteit Leuven
- June 1997: Degree of Medical Doctor, Faculty of Medicine, Katholieke Universiteit Leuven (magna cum laude)
- June 1990: Latin-Sciences Humanities, Abdijschool, Dendermonde

Work experience

- October - September 2006: Clinical attachment at the old age psychiatry section, centre of ageing and mental health sciences, department of mental health sciences, University College London
- Since April 2005: Staff member Psychiatry Department, University Hospitals, Leuven
- August 2004 - march 2005: Resident Psychiatry Department, University Hospitals, Leuven
- October 2002 - September 2006: Research fellow Cognitive Neurology Laboratory, Section Experimental Neurology, K.U. Leuven
- August 2001 - July 2004: Clinical trainee in Psychiatry, University Hospitals, Leuven
- August 2000 - July 2001: Clinical trainee in Psychiatry, Europa Ziekenhuizen, Brussel
- August 1997 - July 2000: Clinical trainee in Surgery, Neurology and Neurosurgery

International Publications

- **M. Vandenbulcke**, R. Peeters, P. Dupont, P. Van Hecke, R. Vandenberghe. Word reading and posterior temporal dysfunction in amnestic mild cognitive impairment. *Cerebral cortex*, 2007; In press.
- J. Theuns, E. Marjaux, **M. Vandenbulcke**, K. Van Laere, S. Kumar-Singh, G. Bormans, M. Van den Broeck, K. Vennekens, E. Corsmit, B. De Strooper, C. Van Broeckhoven, R. Vandenberghe. Alzheimer dementia caused by a novel mutation located furthest C-terminal in APP. *Human Mutation*, 2006; 27: 888-896.

- **M. Vandenbulcke**, R. Peeters, K. Fannes, R. Vandenberghe. Knowledge of visual attributes in the right hemisphere. *Nature Neurosci*, 2006; 9: 964 - 970.

- **M. Vandenbulcke**, R. Peeters, K. Porke, P. Van Hecke, R. Vandenberghe. Anterior temporal rightward laterality in primary progressive aphasia shifts to the right. *Annals of Neurology*, 2005; 58: 362 - 370.

- R. Vandenberghe, **M.Vandenbulcke**, S. Weintraub, N. Johnson, K. Porke, C. Thompson, M. Mesulam. Paradoxical features of word finding difficulty in primary progressive aphasia: Evidence from primed picture naming. *Annals of Neurology*, 2005; 57:204 - 209.

- R. Vandenberghe, S. Geeraerts, P. Molenberghs, C. Lafosse, **M. Vandenbulcke**, K. Peeters, R. Peeters, P. Van Hecke, G.A. Orban. Attentional responses to unattended stimuli in human parietal cortex. *Brain*. 2005; 128:2843 - 2857

- E. Coppens, D. Vansteenwegen, A. Spruyt, **M. Vandenbulcke**, W. Van Paesschen, P. Eelen. Automatice affective stimulus processing is intact after unilateral resection of the anterior temporal lobe in humans *Neuropsychologia*, 2007; In press.

- E. Coppens, D. Vansteenwegen, F. Baeyens, **M. Vandenbulcke**, W. Van Paesschen, P. Eelen. Evaluative conditioning is intact after unilateral resection of the anterior temporal lobe in humans. *Neuropsychologia*, 2006; 44:840 - 843

National Publications

- F. Eeckhout and **M. Vandenbulcke**. Depressie en dementie: een relatie apart. *Tijdschrift voor Geneeskunde*, 2007; In press.

- **M. Vandenbulcke**, J. Janssens. Acute axonal polyneuropathy in chronic alcoholism and malnutrition. *Acta Neurologica Belgica*. 1999; 99(3):198 - 201.

Abstracts

- N. Nelissen, **M. Vandenbulcke**, P. Dupont, R. Peeters, K. Van Laere, G. Bormans, R. Vandenberghe Amyloid deposition and fMRI activity during lexical-semantic retrieval in early stage Alzheimer's disease. Soc. Neurosci. Abs., 2006, 707.8.

- **M. Vandenbulcke**, R. Peeters, K. Porke, P. Van Hecke, R. Vandenberghe Progression of language impairment in Primary Progressive Aphasia: Cognitive and structural MRI predictors. Alzheimer and Dementia, 2006, Vol. 2, Supplement 3, S343.

- N. Nelissen, P. Dupont, **M. Vandenbulcke**, K. Van Laere, G.Bormans, A. Verbruggen, L. Mortelmans, R. Vandenberghe Voxel-wise Analysis of Amyloid Deposition in Early-stage Alzheimer's Disease and Relationship with Cognitive Manifestations. Alzheimer and Dementia, 2006, Vol. 2, Supplement 3, S345 - S346.

- R. Vandenberghe, R. Peeters, P. Van Hecke, **M. Vandenbulcke** Anterior Thalamic Aphasia is Associated with Dysfunction of Left Frontal Operculum and Anterior Inferior Frontal Gyrus. Stroke, 2006, Supplement 1, S49.

- **M. Vandenbulcke**, R. Peeters, P. Van Hecke, R. Vandenberghe Activation of the Visual Word Form Area for words and pictures presented in the left or right visual field. NeuroImage, june, 2005, Vol. 26, Supplement 1, S49.
- R. Vandenberghe, **M.Vandenbulcke**, P. Dupont, R. Peeters, P. Van Hecke fMRI of language and semantic memory in mild cognitive impairment. NeuroImage, june, 2005, Vol. 26, Supplement 1, S48.
- V. Kinnard, P. Dupont, **M. Vandenbulcke**, K. Van Laere, R. Vandenberghe Comparison of kinetic modelling strategies of N-[11C]-Methylpiperidin-4-yl-Proprionate ([11C]-PMP) in normals and patients with Mild Cognitive Impairment (MCI). Journal of Cerebral Blood Flow and Metabolism, 2005, Vol. 25, S593.
- **M. Vandenbulcke**, R. Peeters, P. Van Hecke, R. Vandenberghe. Activation of the visual word form area for words and pictures presented in the left or right visual field. Soc. Neurosci. Abs., 2004.
- R. Vandenberghe, **M. Vandenbulcke**, R. Peeters, P. Van Hecke. Ageing and the meaning of words and pictures. Soc. Neurosci. Abs., 2004, 14.3.
- R. Vandenberghe, **M. Vandenbulcke**, P. Dupont, G. Bormans, A. Verbruggen, L. Mortelmans, K. Van Laere. Voxel-based parametric mapping of acetylcholinesterase activity using [11C]-PMP in mild cognitive impairment. ANA (American Neurological Association), 2004.
- R. Vandenberghe, **M. Vandenbulcke**, R. Peeters, K. Porke, P. Van Hecke, R. Vandenberghe. Associative semantics with words and pictures in Mild Cognitive Impairment. Neurobiology of Aging, july, 2004, Vol. 25, S2, p S278.
- **M. Vandenbulcke**, R. Peeters, K. Porke, P. Van Hecke, R. Vandenberghe. Right anterior temporal activity during word and picture semantics in Primary Progressive Aphasia. Neurobiology of Aging, july, 2004 Vol. 25,S2, p S277.
- K. Van Laere, **M. Vandenbulcke**, P. Dupont, G. Bormans, A. Verbruggen, L. Mortelmans, R. Vandenberghe. Voxel-based parametric mapping of acetylcholinesterase activity using [11C]-PMP in mild cognitive impairment. European Association of Nuclear Medicine, Helsinki, 2004.
- R. Peeters, **M. Vandenbulcke**, R. Vandenberghe, P. Van Hecke . Visualizing anterior temporal activation during semantic processing with parallel imaging techniques. Twelfth scientific meeting and exhibition of the ISMRM, 15-20 may 2004, Kyoto Japan, pp.739.
- R. Vandenberghe, **M. Vandenbulcke**, S. Geeraerts, R. Peeters, P. Van Hecke. Extinction-like brain response to bilateral simultaneous stimulation in normal subjects. Soc. Neurosci. Abs., 2003, 228.12.
- **M. Vandenbulcke**, R. Peeters, P. Van Hecke, R. Vandenberghe. Right fusiform activation during semantic processing of pictures. Soc. Neurosci. Abs., 2003, 770.7.

Awards

Award from the National Institute of Mental Health of the NIH (Award # 2 R13 MH062008-06, "Conference on Functional Mapping of the Human Brain").